ALSO BY ELISABETH HASSELBECK

The G-Free Diet: A Gluten-Free Survival Guide

Deliciously
G-Free

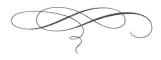

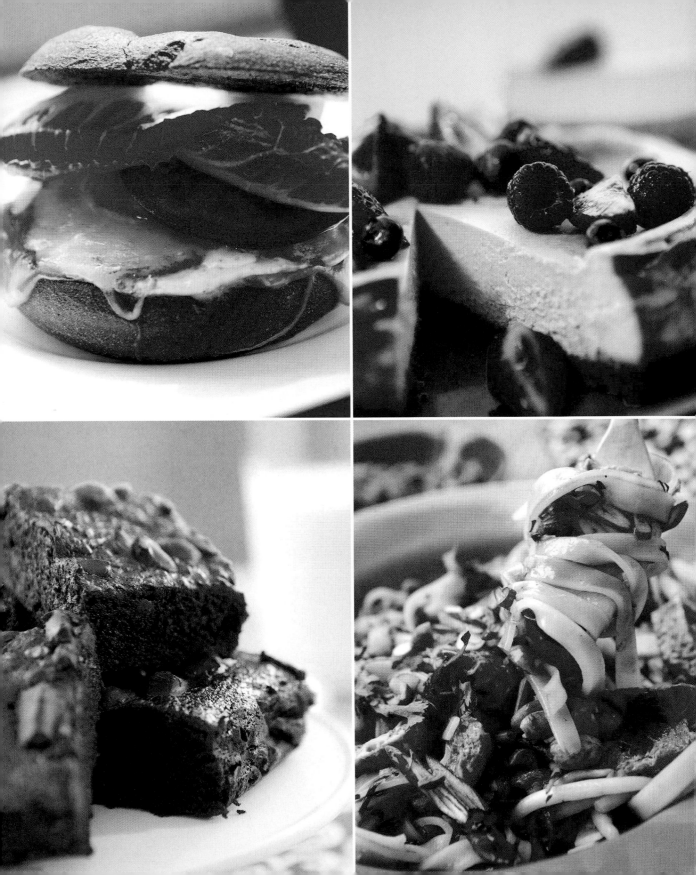

Deliciously G-Free

FOOD SO FLAVORFUL THEY'LL
NEVER BELIEVE IT'S GLUTEN-FREE

Elisabeth Hasselbeck

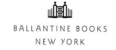

BALLANTINE BOOKS
NEW YORK

Copyright © 2012 by Elisabeth Hasselbeck Enterprises, LLC

Photographs copyright © 2012 by Kelly Campbell

Published in the United States by Ballantine Books, an imprint of The Random House Publishing Group, a division of Random House, Inc., New York.

BALLANTINE and colophon are registered trademarks of Random House, Inc.

Library of Congress Cataloging-in-Publication Data

Hasselbeck, Elisabeth.
Deliciously g-free : food so flavorful they'll never believe it's gluten-free / Elisabeth Hasselbeck.
p. cm.
Includes index.
ISBN 978-0-345-52938-1 (hardback)—ISBN 978-0-345-52940-4 (ebook)
1. Gluten-free diet—Recipes. I. Title.
RM237.86.H368 2012
641.3—dc23
2011035301

Printed in the United States of America on acid-free paper

www.ballantinebooks.com

2 4 6 8 9 7 5 3 1

First Edition

Book design by Diane Hobbing

To Grace, Taylor, and Isaiah
I love you with my whole heart

{ Contents }

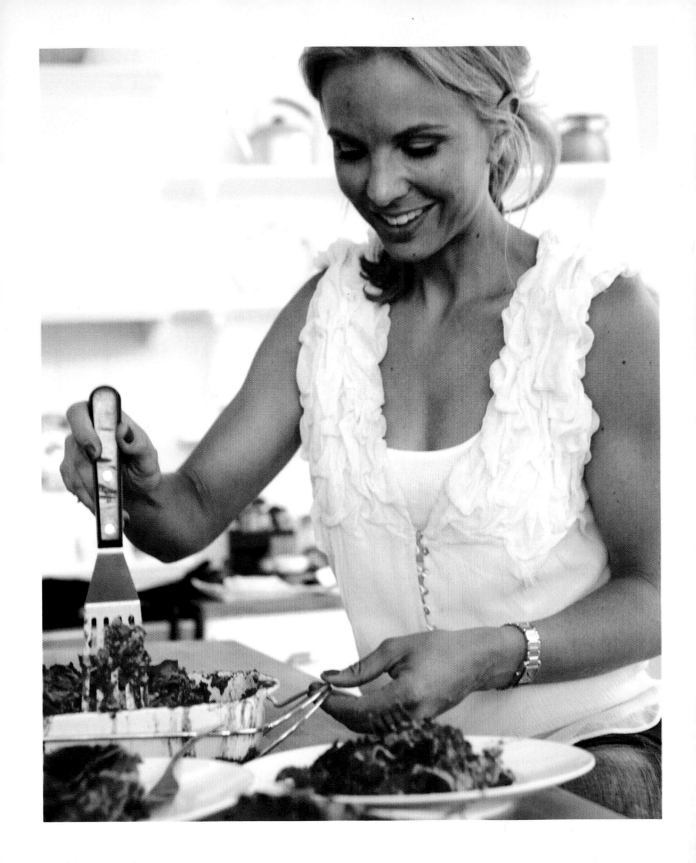

A Culinary Homecoming

"Mommy, are you remembering what it was like when you were a little girl?" my daughter, Grace, asked while we sat at the dinner table, my eyes closed as I savored a g-free version of my grandmother's meatballs. Happily, I was—finally! Thanks to my mom, who had been working with me to adapt and perfect that long-loved recipe for my gluten-free needs, for the first time it tasted just like Mama's (as we called my grandmother). It was in that moment that the desire to write this cookbook was born, and the direction clear: rediscovering the foods I once loved but had lost for too long, due to my celiac disease. It was time to bring back timelessly delicious food, but deliciously g-free for the first time.

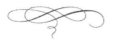

I grew up in the heart of an Italian-American neighborhood in Providence, Rhode Island. Our apartment was on the third floor, and my great-grandmother, who had come from Italy to America at the young age of sixteen and whom we called Mama Great, lived on the first floor. She was the last person to see us out the door in the morning, and the first to see us come home. No matter what the time was on the clock, her kitchen always smelled as if dinner was just moments away. The concrete sidewalks outside the apartment building hid a lush backyard garden—like "a pearl in an oyster," as my mom always says—where we grew eggplant, tomatoes, basil, and green beans, all of which made their way to our family table. Snapping fresh green beans from their stems was just one of my many "jobs" (I hired myself!). Later in the season there were clusters of fragrant deep purple grapes to pick from the homemade trellis (which seemed like a huge vineyard when we were kids) and pop from their skins. Mama Great also had a basement full of treasures: homemade pepper biscuits, wine, and jelly. Straight from the school bus, I'd knock first on her door if I smelled biscuits in the oven. I knew that she might need me to "paint" them with egg wash to make them shiny.

Just minutes away by car, and years later a five-mile run, lived my mom's mom, "Mama." Her thumb was so green, I still think she could grow anything out of plain dirt! We kids spent many afternoons carrying as many plum tomatoes or zucchini as possible into the house. Mama's house was everyone's home.

Mama was most often at the stove tending a large pot that was almost overflowing with meatballs and sauce. We grandkids would try to be patient for the two perfectly browned meatballs she'd hand to each of us when they were ready. She kept track of how many she made and was proud to give us the final number every time. On big feast holidays or for special events, she made so many as to be almost uncountable. Later, when I was on the softball team at Boston College and we were passing through Rhode Island, Mama made the whole team a meal, with a record seventy-two meatballs!

Meals were special in my home. We never rushed, and the food and great (loud) conversation kept our family at the table for hours. At every major holiday, Mama made a Big Dish—baked macaroni and lasagna were the two I remember best. On Thanksgiving, even the turkey was a side dish to Mama's main event. "Isn't it beautiful!" everyone would say as she brought the dish to the table. She would beam. It was oh-so-good to eat, but more important, the beauty was that Mama honored us with her specialty and that she, in turn, felt honored when we ate it so enthusiastically.

Enter . . . the Italian bread. A thirty-inch-long fresh-baked loaf was a staple at every meal, there to soak up every last drop of sauce or salad dressing and even to be dipped into coffee at the end. Some of the best conversations were had over "coffee and," as we called it. To this day, the meals end with this, and the next morning, the bread is toasted and buttered for breakfast.

As we grew older, my parents kept alive the traditional meals of their childhoods as well. My mom continued the tradition of stuffed peppers, baked macaroni, and biscuits. My dad's Polish heritage brought kielbasa, gwumpkies (stuffed cabbage rolls), and pierogies. After decades of taking for granted the meals that we had growing up, I am now a working mom myself, and I remain in awe of my parents' ability to work all day and still put something so good on the table at night. My father, a brilliant architect, has also become quite the creative chef and he never disappoints when it comes to food presentation. My mom, who initially taught high school biology and chemistry, made a career change shortly after my brother was born, when I was just over two years old. She found her calling in law, and she went back to school for her degree at night, taking the bus from Providence to Boston for her classes. I remember going along for the ride to the bus stop in my footie pajamas. My parents' commitment to their careers never interfered with their devotion to putting our family first, and somehow they both managed to continue to bring us together with home-cooked family meals.

I still ask my mom at least once a week how she did it all. "We just did!" she says. And every week that passes, I understand that response more and more. It is a challenge for any parent, working or not, to get it together for dinnertime. There are days when I am at the stove with my kids running in and out of the kitchen (sometimes offering to "help," which isn't always so helpful!), hungry bellies leading to whines and sibling battles, and I think,

"Why didn't I just order pizza?" Indeed, the witching hour of dinner preparation is never picture-perfect. But the result—sitting together and talking over a meal (even on pizza delivery nights)—is just that: perfect.

My mom is always sharing her tips, and one of them is to embrace the freezer. Defrosting something you made earlier still counts as a home-cooked meal in my book! I never feel guilty reheating quality food that I made myself, freezer burn and all. Time and again, devoting one or two days to cooking and freezing has made all the difference for me later in the week. Using this strategy, I am able to maintain the home-cooked vibe without losing my mind. If I had it my way, I would always have the time, the space, the groceries lined up, and every ingredient on hand to make every meal for everyone. Reality check: I don't. But putting in a couple evenings of cooking from my repertoire of easy-to-make and yummy gluten-free main meals, side dishes, and goodies has become my best strategy. Make a super batch of g-free Mama's meatballs, or chicken soup, or chicken tenders, and cupcakes—all easily frozen—and I am golden for the week! Serving something hot out of the oven the same day I make it feels great. Knowing that I have made enough to extend to a second or even third meal is nothing short of liberating.

Being busy *and* gluten-free might have meant that my family traditions would fade, but developing the recipes in this book and cooking from them regularly allows us all to continue to eat our favorite foods. And for me, that has meaning beyond words.

There was a time when I was certain that neither of those two obstacles would be overcome. After I realized that I had celiac disease, I was sidelined at the family table. I missed the obvious deliciousness of Mama's treats, but also I missed partaking in the celebration of what she had worked on all day. Mama was sad every time I passed the platter along without taking a helping for myself. "What do you mean you can't have the ziti?" she would exclaim, concerned that I was not getting what she knew was too good to pass up. And for nearly a decade, I would sorely attempt to explain. But back then, celiac disease wasn't as understood or accepted as it is today, and Mama had a hard time believing that a good Italian girl couldn't eat her pasta. There were even times when I would eat the food anyway, fully aware that I'd pay for it in the short term with serious stomach pain, and in the long run with damage to my intestine and immune system. Seeing her dimpled smile, having her content to be watching me eat something she'd made with her whole heart, made it worth it.

Outside of Mama's house, however, gluten was no longer a part of my diet. In 2008, after nearly a decade of learning to live gluten-free the hard way, I wrote *The G-Free Diet*. My goal: to let everyone else in on all that I had experienced—from initial misdiagnosis to finally obtaining a proper diagnosis of celiac disease, from ordering in, dining out, and being a guest in someone else's home to shopping the aisles of a grocery store with an eye toward hidden gluten.

Of course, food is more than an energy source or the experience of taste. It's a social catalyst, a thing that can bring people together, as it had in my childhood. During my transition to becoming totally g-free, however, food seemed to be the enemy and I couldn't enjoy the social element of sharing it with others. I basically went from food-loving to food-fearing. The communal table seemed more like the "cubicle table," with the meals looking as if everyone had ordered something different from the menu. I was hungry for good food—flavorful, memorable, delicious—but I was also starving for the connectedness to my family and my heritage.

Ultimately, this cookbook was born out of my deep desire to make great food that I can eat and that everyone (whether you have celiac disease, a gluten intolerance, or are g-free for any other great reason) can enjoy! I am finally at the point where I can make dishes from my childhood or my husband's, and we *all* (including our three kids) absolutely love them. Whether you come to this book because of your own or a loved one's gluten sensitivity or because you've heard about the wonderful health or energy benefits of going gluten-free, my dearest hope is that you too will find joy and flavor again in cooking this way. With a wide variety of gluten-free ingredients now on the market, and by learning to use other wonderful and tasty binders in your cooking, there's simply no reason to settle for something (as I once did) because it is the only option. Uninteresting and uninspired gluten-free cooking is a thing of the past! Deliciously G-Free Cuisine is here!

In the process of testing recipes and looking for ingredients that are gluten-free and free of cross-contamination (more on that later—it is an important concern), I've become my own g-free chef. The real seal of approval comes to me in the form of "Wow, so good! May I have more of that?" or "Yummy, Mommy. Can we have this again tomorrow?" Full disclosure: Many a time I have had to learn the hard way—but with this book, I pass along my tips, shortcuts, and ideas so you can lose your fear of the unknown and get back to happy eating and sharing some great dishes. Welcome back, flavor and variety!

It is with thankfulness that I am able to pass these recipes on to my own children and to you, my deliciously g-free kitchenistas!

And now . . . let the fun begin!

Deliciously
G-Free

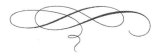

{Chapter 1}

The G-Free Kitchen

Celiac disease is a digestive disorder characterized by a toxic reaction to gluten, the protein found in certain grains. An autoimmune condition (meaning it causes the body to attack itself, dramatically weakening the body's ability to ward off infections and other disease), celiac disease is hereditary and chronic. It's *not* a food allergy, and for those with celiac, avoiding gluten completely is the only way to live (literally). The cure: G-FREE food.

According to researchers at the University of Chicago, 1 in 133 people have celiac disease—meaning 3 million Americans alone! The problem is, only 1 percent of those with it have received a diagnosis. The rest of the pack likely lives with chronic, inexplicable abdominal pain, low energy, and a host of other symptoms. Thankfully, in the past five years, diagnosis has improved (thanks to great physicians like Dr. Peter Green, who not only diagnosed me but has devoted his career to treating patients as well as educating those in his field in order to properly flag and test for the disease) and labeling on foods is more accurate, allowing those with celiac to navigate the g-free world more easily.

Though not classified as a disease, gluten sensitivity (sometimes called non-celiac gluten sensitivity, or gluten intolerance) affects an approximate 6 percent of the American population, causing digestive aggravation when gluten is ingested. With improvements to testing for these conditions and education in the medical establishment, more and more people are getting clear diagnoses and are beginning to go in search of gluten-free foods.

The community of those eating g-free is therefore expanding, and we are hungry!

I wrote in great detail of the roadblocks I faced in my own journey to diagnosis, and the tips and strategies I learned as I began to eat food that would not make me sick, in my first book, *The G-Free Diet*. To this day, I hear from people from all walks of life—moms, dads, friends, colleagues, and even strangers on the street—who tell me that *The G-Free Diet* is a friend to them, an easy reference to navigating the proverbial food waters g-free style.

Whether you have celiac or gluten sensitivity (or even if you simply want to stop eating gluten for other health or energy reasons), your goals are to replace glutenous grains with more impactful, less harmful gluten-free grains; to avoid any kind of cross-contamination in your kitchen (and be on guard for it in restaurants and at parties); and to effectively and confidently communicate your food situation to those around you.

Creating a safe cooking haven for yourself—a completely g-free kitchen—will meet those goals. Living with a completely g-free kitchen will mean that any crumbs are not immediately suspect, and it'll mean less double washing and cleaning!

If this change is just not possible for you—perhaps you are aiming to please a houseful of non-g-free-ers in addition to your own needs—what I call "the hybrid kitchen" will be more your style. In my own home, I'd say we currently have a 60 percent g-free kitchen, though every day the percentage is growing as we find more and more products (and develop them, too) that are safe for my sensitive digestive system.

The initial step of g-freeing your kitchen to whatever extent you are able will pay big dividends in the end. The more g-free your kitchen, the less stress you will have when addressing cross-contamination. Simple steps have made food preparation a lot less worrisome for me—and they will for you, too.

Elisabeth Hasselbeck

STORING G-FREE PRODUCTS

I recently went into a coffee shop that sold g-free treats. The problem, though, was that they were on the shelf *below* the gluten-containing muffins, which rained crumbs all over the supposedly g-free offerings every time one was pulled out.

With this in mind, think of anything with gluten like a leaking pen. Anything that it travels over will be "inked." Therefore, one of the most important considerations in a hybrid kitchen is *where* you store your products. If you can't dedicate a whole cabinet to g-free ingredients alone, you can still avoid gluten contamination by following this handy rule of thumb: Gluten "goes low" and g-free "flies high." That is, store your g-free products *above* the others. If you were to store gluten above g-free, you would run the risk of crumbs from gluten products falling into the g-free packaging or containers, as they did in that coffee shop.

Here's another rule of thumb: On a buffet, place g-free dishes first and in the front, and gluten options last and in the back. This way, there is less "fly-over," less possibility that gluten options will drip into or fall onto the g-free platters as people make their way down the line.

> When setting up your hybrid g-free kitchen, remember my rule of thumb: Gluten goes low, g-free flies high! On a buffet, avoid "fly-over" contamination by placing g-free platters and dishes where your family and guests will serve themselves first.

Cool Storage

In my home, the refrigerator is already a mostly gluten-free zone, without our having to try too hard to make it so. Fresh foods (like vegetables, fruits, meats, dairy, and herbs) are naturally gluten-free, and most of our jarred foods and condiments long ago got a g-free makeover (everything from ketchup to mayo and syrups and flavorings now come in g-free brands) because having two of everything overcrowded the fridge. For products that we go through quickly, like peanut butter and jelly, we do stock both options, but I use labels on the g-free versions so that a knife that just made the trip across a piece of whole wheat bread does not go for a dip in my g-free jar.

As with the kitchen cabinets, I keep the non-g-free foods on the bottom shelf of the fridge so that if anything falls, drips, or spills out of a gluten-containing leftover or soupy dish, it does not travel over the items that are g-free. If g-free offerings will be in the minority in your fridge, keep them in a plastic tub (also labeled) to protect them from the g-full food.

Space permitting, many g-free families find that a small, dedicated "g-free-zer" is a huge time- and worry-saver. Try storing a supply of deliciously g-free cupcakes (pages 194–198), muffins (pages 43–48), g-free pizza dough (page 170), the double batch of chicken fingers (page 83), and cookie dough (page 215) this way. At a minimum, I recommend that you set aside a section of your freezer for non-g-free foods just the way you did in your fridge. Be sure to use the location rules, and keep your breaded non-g-free chicken tenders or nuggets below or behind the g-free versions.

Elisabeth Hasselbeck

Dry Storage

Once you start cooking from the recipes in this book, I hope you will feel that g-free flours, pastas, and flavorings are just as good as, if not *better than*, the gluten-heavy versions you might now have in your pantry. As g-free replacements begin to take up greater real estate in your kitchen, you might actually be looking to donate the boxes of pasta, unopened bags of flour, and a whole range of other ingredients that you just don't need around anymore! Or you might be inclined to have a "going away party" for your glutenous goodies: a big bakeoff and last hoorah.

Even if you're not giving your gluten products away entirely, when creating a hybrid kitchen it's a good idea to make a fresh start with your pantry. Opened bags of flour or boxes of pasta can rain potential contaminants onto your shelves and into the cracks and corners between them. Give your pantry, cupboards, and silverware drawers a thorough "spring cleaning," wiping them out with soap and hot water. For safe measure, put all your silverware and cooking utensils through a sanitizing dishwasher cycle, too.

Think about the crumbs that find their way into your cooking utensil or silverware drawers. Go ahead—I dare you to take a look right now! It's amazing how many crumbs congregate there, isn't it? You may not have the flexibility in your kitchen to move your silverware and utensils to a spot away from where food is prepared, but *do* strive to place your breadbox somewhere other than over your utensil drawer (and don't store any glutenous snacks on top of where the drawer opens). This will dramatically cut down on any possible contamination to the silverware and utensils you rely on, and it's one of the most effective (and easy) g-free steps you can take.

> In our house, the breadbox is where we keep glutenous items—bread, baked goods—because it's a way to keep them separate from the rest of the kitchen. I happen to give my g-free baked goods the prime display space: a glass-covered cake dish on my counter! For extended storage, I place g-free breads and baked treats in the freezer or fridge. Whatever you decide to do, the key is to be consistent: explain the new system to the family, babysitters, houseguests, etc., and stick to it!

Be Loud and Clear

Once you've decided on your organizational system, do yourself the big favor of labeling containers and cookware (including knives, if one will be used for cutting or spreading with exclusively g-free foods) in a way that will remind the family to stick with the program. Use a label maker, a brand of labels that really adhere (I like Mabel's Labels or Stuck on You labels, which stick even when they go through a dishwasher), or a Sharpie pen, so that there's no confusion about what is g-free. Label drawers, shelves, bags of flours, jars of peanut butter and mayo. If there is a label on it, everyone will know that it is gluten-free. What a worry-saver for you, the person trying to avoid gluten altogether! Here are some other handy tips for setting up and working in a hybrid kitchen:

- Dishcloths, sponges, and scrubbers are hiding places for gluten if they've been used to clean up after a gluten meal. Keep a g-free set of them in a designated spot.
- Even if you've designated several sponges or scrubbers for g-free use, run them through the dishwasher every time it cycles to banish g-crumbs and buildup that may have come through exposure to gluten food.
- Develop a simple system for wiping down the countertop

Elisabeth Hasselbeck

before cooking your evening meal. Use soap and hot water, and the sponge or cloth that you've designated for g-free use. Better safe than sorry. If you have celiac disease, it takes only ⅛ teaspoon of gluten a day to damage the intestine. Every crumb counts.

- Paper towels are the unsung hero of any kitchen—think about how often you use them!—but nowhere more so than in the hybrid kitchen. If you don't know which dishcloth or sponge is the g-free one, grab a paper towel for a fast and effective wipe down or hand drying.

- Be sure to inspect the ingredients in the soap and hand lotion you keep by your kitchen sink to make sure that there is no gluten in them. Think about it: If you wash or moisturize your hands (or both) and then turn your attention to, say, making a salad, you may well be contaminating the lettuce with the trace gluten on your hands.

READY, SET, COOK!

Okay, your kitchen is clean, organized, and ready to go. You want to get down to business, so what about cooking equipment? There is no need to invest in a whole new set of cookware to set your kitchen up for g-free gourmet goodness, but there are a few things to consider for safety.

Plastic

Plastic can trap gluten if it is badly scratched and really worn. Relegate scratched plastic containers to the gluten cabinet or invest in a set of glass storage containers that will last a lifetime and can easily be washed if something with gluten does mistakenly get stored in them. If you don't choose to label your containers as g-free and gluten-allowed, use two sets with different-colored tops to make the difference clear for everyone.

Baking Pans and Baking Sheets

If you have an old family pie dish or cake pan—inherited from your grandmother's kitchen, perhaps—there is a fast and simple solution to continuing to use it in your gluten-free cooking: line pie dishes or cake pans with aluminum foil, and spread parchment paper or foil over the baking sheet. Since cupcakes and muffins are regularly requested at my house (and since I find that cookies tend to stick to foil, even when it's greased), I have a designated and completely g-free muffin tin, and to avoid mishaps I also have two designated g-free baking sheets.

> Since my diagnosis with celiac disease, I have been steadily building up a g-free set of kitchen items. My wish list for birthdays always includes a "double" of something I've had in my kitchen since Tim and I got married: a pot, a pan, a mixing bowl, a set of knives, a cutting board. This is a slow but steady way to duplicate the basic equipment we've been using, and a good way to substitute g-free items as the older ones get scuffed, stained, and cracked.

Stainless Steel

One hundred percent stainless steel pots and pans are a go! I recommend scrubbing them well with plenty of dishwashing soap and then also running them through the dishwasher before considering them a part of your g-free tool set.

Glass

Glass is a nonporous surface, so once they are really clean, glass bowls and bakeware will be a great asset to you. They are great for mixing, measuring, and baking. Glass baking dishes tend to conduct heat faster than metal, though, so to avoid dry baked goods, be careful with recommended cook times. My mom usually made brownies in a Pyrex dish—the smooth surface is so easy to clean—and so do I.

Nonstick

Some nonstick surfaces like Teflon may trap gluten if they are damaged and/or not washed properly. I use ceramic-lined pans for a healthier nonstick surface. Investing in one large ceramic-lined frying pan for recipes like chicken fingers (page 85), and one small one for eggs, like the omelet (page 31) and frittata (page 35), is ideal. Of course, if your entire kitchen is g-free, and not hybrid, any pan you have will work.

Utensils and Knives

Just like stainless steel pots and pans, stainless steel utensils are safe if they are properly cleaned. Stainless steel knives are a must and are very durable; an 8-inch chef's knife and one or two paring knives are all you'll need for the recipes in this book. If you already own stainless steel knives, just be sure to take extra time to clean around the handle and hilt to be sure no food particles linger in any crevices.

A flexible high-heat nylon or silicone spatula is a great, inexpensive addition to your gluten-free utensil drawer and will make flipping eggs and pancakes easier. (Sometimes they can be a little too floppy, though, so select one that you can maneuver well.)

Even if you clean them out regularly, your toaster and toaster oven un-doubtedly harbor bread crumbs. Though this will take up precious counter space, I highly recommend designating a special toaster and toaster oven as g-free in your hybrid kitchen.

GETTING DELICIOUSLY STOCKED

Many of my recipes are centered around easy-to-find, naturally gluten-free ingredients like vegetables, fruits, meats, dairy, whole grains, and herbs. Now that gluten-free baking has become more popular, g-free flours like brown rice, tapioca, and potato flours are readily available in large supermarkets, in health food stores, and online. See my tips for g-free baking on page 15 to learn more about the products I think taste and cook up best.

Food manufacturers are finding ways to improve the texture and taste of g-free breads every day. In the case of gluten-free pastas, many that are already on the market taste so good that everyone can enjoy a big bowl of g-free pasta topped with an amazing Bolognese Sauce (page 114) or Spanish Chicken (page 109), or even as a base for my kid-friendly Mac and Cheese (page 175). Of course, *quality* replacement is key, so buy small boxes or packages of g-free staples to determine which brand you like best.

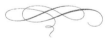

Thanks to more comprehensive and much more visible g-free (GF) labeling, shopping for great gluten-free options is the easiest it has ever been. There are still some items that can throw you for a loop, though, so be prepared to keep an eye out for these:

Elisabeth Hasselbeck

Butter

Butter is one of those luscious, rich, chef-friendly items that makes it onto every gluten-free shopping list. But some brands of "unsalted" or "sweet" butters have "natural flavorings" on their ingredient list. What exactly is a "natural flavoring"? Well, it can be one of a host of ingredients processed from a natural food source, including essences, oils, proteins, and, yes, grains. Some natural flavorings are even derived from hydrolyzed wheat and barley. That's why I call for *salted* butter in the recipes—and to balance out the salt, I simply scale down the amount of table or sea salt I would normally add. Salted butters usually don't contain "natural flavorings," but be on the safe side and check the label before you make your purchase.

Bacon

Just like butter, bacon is close to the heart of great home cooks and chefs alike. Most smoke flavorings are produced by burning hardwoods and gathering their condensation. However, some smoke flavorings can contain yeast, which means there is a chance there could be trace amounts of gluten in the bacon. Thankfully, there are still many brands of bacon that are traditionally wood-smoked. Be sure to check the label of the brand you buy.

Sour Cream

Most whole sour creams on the market are gluten-free, but "light" sour creams can be thickened with flours, starches, and stabilizers that can be hidden havens for gluten. I recommend going for the full-fat option and then lightening up the fat content in other ways, such as using less oil or opting for a g-free cooking spray.

Meat and Vegetable Broths

Whether they are in cans or cartons, most meat and vegetable broths have a long list of mystery ingredients that will make your head spin. You'll see ingredients like "natural flavorings," hydrolyzed protein (which can come from wheat bran and other gluten-containing ingredients), and autolyzed yeast extract used as a binder (which can be derived from brewer's yeast and often contains MSG). This was something that tripped me up many a time in restaurants that used a stock to cook items like rice or meats. Even when I first began cooking g-free, I would inadvertently make myself sick by making chili with a base that had gluten in it. Finding out the hard way was never fun! I opt for broths that clearly state "gluten free" on the label. I also periodically do a check of manufacturer websites to see if they are clear and up front about their manufacturing process. I'm also on the lookout for Internet chatter about less than 100 percent adherence to g-free preparation. (See page 92 for my chicken broth recipe.)

Brown Sugar

Brown sugar is traditionally processed raw sugar that is made soft and fragrant by retaining some of the syrup released in the initial heating process. Some brown sugars are also glazed with a small percentage of iron-rich molasses to enhance texture and color. So far, so good.

However, some food companies use caramel flavoring in place of molasses to give brown sugar its characteristic golden-brown hue. Caramel colorings are produced by heating carbohydrates—wheat among them—and many classes of these colorings are used in everything from beer to candy. To be safe, look for brown sugar without "caramel flavoring" in the ingredient list. As with any questionable item, I strongly recommended contacting the manufacturer to check the source of the ingredients.

Elisabeth Hasselbeck

THE SECRETS OF G-FREE BAKING

Over the years, gluten-free baking has been hit-or-miss with me, from spectacular and over-the-top to a crumbly bust. But *your* worries are over because I have ironed out all the wrinkles for you! With the hard work behind me, I am handing over the play-book on the substitutes for gluten, on how the gluten-free flours work, recipes for making your own flour mixes, and tips on making the ultimate tender baked goods that even kids will give a "thumbs-up" to.

To be sure I have the flavors just right, I gave the ultimate taste-test to my husband, close friends, and family, all of whom never used to eat g-free. They are the ones who needed to be convinced that what they were eating tasted just like, or even better than, the glutenous competition. If I could get someone who did not *need* to eat g-free to love something that *was*, I'd know I'd found sweet success! The proof is literally in the pudding (page 206), in my devil's food cupcakes with chocolate buttercream icing (page 197), and in the perfect, buttery chocolate chip cookie (page 215) that will even have the toughest cookie connoisseur sneaking seconds!

Substitutes for Gluten

Gluten is a combination of two binding proteins, gliadin and glutenin. Found in wheat, rye, and barley—the very ingredients to avoid on a g-free diet—these proteins are what give bread its chewy bounce and cakes and brownies their delicate, moist crumb. Without gluten, or without the major players that step in to do its work, most baked goods crumble and lack that tender, moist, or chewy texture that makes homemade treats so good. Xanthan gum and guar gum have been pinch-hitting for gluten in baking for some time. If you've done any g-free baking up to this point, you've probably encountered them in recipe ingredient lists. But if you've not heard of them before, don't be intimidated! Here's what you need to know:

Xanthan gum is a binder made from the fermentation of sugars isolated from corn. Traditionally it is used in salad dressings to help them pour well and prevent separation, and it is added to toothpaste and ice creams to help those products maintain their thick, mousselike consistency. (If you've ever had xanthan gum clinging to your fingertips, then washed your hands, you've noticed an interesting slippery film forming on your fingers before it melts away.) In baked goods, xanthan gum increases the viscosity of the batter. Xanthan gum is sold in powder form, usually in 5- to 6-ounce bags. Since it's used in small amounts, one bag will be enough to supply you with great baked goods for many months to come.

Guar gum is derived from the seed of a plant grown in India and is typically found in powder form (like xanthan gum) in health food and specialty food stores. Guar gum has eight times the thickening power of standard starches, like corn or potato, and gives more bounce to baked goods. Commercially, it's used for a thickener in hot and cold drinks, and you'll find it in your favorite summertime Popsicles.

Both xanthan and guar gum range wildly in price—from $3.50 a bag to $12 per 8 ounces, depending on where you buy it. Look for deals on the Internet, but remember that there's no need to order either one in bulk since most baked goods require only a teaspoon.

Elisabeth Hasselbeck

Before you buy, be certain that the company is clear about the gluten-free status, that their xanthan or guar gum isn't processed on or with any equipment that also handles gluten.

In recipes, xanthan and guar gum add the binding and moisturizing properties that are lost without the gluten from wheat, rye, and barley. In most cases you can use xanthan or guar gum interchangeably in cakes, cookies, and breakfast foods like pancakes and waffles. Using too much will create a gummy, almost rubbery baked good, and using too little will mean crumble city—that dry texture that gives g-free baked goods a bad rap. As a rule of thumb, start with 1 teaspoon xanthan or guar gum when converting your favorite traditional cookie or cake recipe.

Just like the g-free flours, xanthan gum and guar gum store well in a dark, cool place. Xanthan gum has a long shelf life, up to two years, and guar gum up to eighteen months, so once you stock your baking shelf, you'll have a go-to ingredient any time you're craving brownies or chocolate chip cookies warm from the oven. I usually mark the date of purchase somewhere on the container, to eliminate guesswork later on.

Power Flour

During one of my first g-free baking trials years ago, I made what was supposed to be a muffin but turned out to be a "sort of scone." Exasperated, I wondered why I had spent so long in the kitchen working to make something that, at best, my husband would eat only out of fear that I might just totally melt down in defeat (I just love him!). The answer: the all-purpose g-free flour I had used. Yuck.

After trying and tasting every combination possibly known to g-free-ers, I have concluded that the best baked goods come from the flours that I mix up myself.

I know what you're thinking: this sounds hard, and all-purpose g-free flour sounds so easy! I agree, but when you invest your time in baking, and you want to indulge yourself and your loved ones, the flavor is crucial. Believe me: you can't afford *not* to make your own flour mixes, and if you follow the easy mix-ahead directions below, all your baked goods will be a snap. Don't waste time on options that are not going to deliver deliciously.

Gluten-free flours are made from whole, naturally gluten-free grains and seeds that are ground into flour. Each flour has its own unique health profile, texture, flavor, and reactive properties during baking. All of the flours mentioned here are available in health food stores and at discounted prices when ordered on the Internet.

Black Bean Flour

Black bean flour works great with dense chocolate desserts because the rich taste of chocolate masks the flavor of the beans. Since beans are high in fiber (a nutritional plus for celiacs), black bean flour holds moisture in chocolate cakes and is a key ingredient in my brownie recipe (page 209). I don't recommend this flour for vanilla-flavored baked goods since the color and bean flavor will come through.

Brown Rice Flour

I consider this the "all-purpose" flour for g-free baking. It has a mild flavor and is a great base for many recipes. Because it has a gritty, slightly granular texture, mix it with flours that are good at absorbing moisture, like black bean, coconut, and sorghum.

Coconut Flour

This is one of my favorite flours. It's extremely high in fiber: just 2 tablespoons deliver 5 grams, a boon for celiac sufferers, who need to supplement their fiber intake. Even if you're not a fan of coconut, mixing small quantities of this golden-yellow flour with other flours improves the texture of your cakes and cupcakes and helps ensure a moist crumb. Coconut flour gives my classic yellow cupcakes (page 194) their lemony color and cuts the graininess of brown rice flour while keeping moisture in.

Millet Flour

Millet flour is milled from a small grain that reminds me of tiny round popcorn kernels, but with a milder yet nutty flavor and a much lighter texture. Since some gluten-free flours don't absorb as much liquid as their glutenous counterparts, millet's drier, chalky consistency and medium texture make it the perfect sponge for any baked good containing moist fruit or large amounts of heavy liquid, like my banana bread (page 213).

Potato Flour

Like coconut flour, potato flour grabs moisture, but it contains less than half the amount of fiber found in coconut flour. It works well when combined with gritty flours like brown rice and sweet white rice to balance out the texture in cookie recipes and baked goods that contain less liquid. Use potato flour in moderation when mixing with other flours, as it burns easily.

Potato Starch

Many g-free bakers say that potato flour and potato starch are the same, but potato starch tends to be a lot finer in consistency and bright white in color, compared to the dull off-white of potato flour. Potato starch works well to enrich sauces and provides a crisp-on-the-outside, soft-inside texture for waffles.

Sweet Sorghum Flour

Sorghum is grain harvested from a grass, and is America's third-largest grain crop. Like gluten-full whole wheat flour, sweet sorghum flour has a dark, speckled cinnamon appearance and a coarse texture. It has a unique mineral profile that is high in iron (for healthy blood and heart), potassium (crucial for hydration), and phosphorus (important for growing bones and teeth). It's the perfect base for quick breads, muffins, pancakes, and biscuits.

Sweet White Rice Flour

Sweet white rice flour reminds me of powdery white cake flour, traditionally used to create the fine crumb for which dainty white cakes are famous. I use sweet rice flour as the main flour in my brownies because, much like cake flour, it has a lighter texture and is higher in starch than brown rice flour. It also seems to magnify the flavor and mimic the texture of the melted chocolate.

Tapioca Starch

Tapioca starch has the lightest, finest texture of all the baking flours. It's responsible for that irresistible "crackle" on top of my brownies (page 209). It also makes the dreamy-smooth pudding filling that you'll find in recipes like my banana cream pie (page 202), and it helps to crisp the outside of my signature chocolate chip cookies (page 215).

Elisabeth Hasselbeck

Some grains may be gluten-free, but they are not invited to my baked-goods party. Here is who they are and why:

Amaranth flour is made from the seed of the amaranth plant, which is cultivated in South America. Although amaranth is a healthy grain, high in protein and amino acids, it has a grassy flavor that tends to dominate the flavor of baked goods, and it also tends to make them crumbly.

Teff flour is milled from an incredibly small seed and has a nutty flavor and dark hue. Much like amaranth, teff has a healthy and unique nutritional profile, high in iron and fiber. Unfortunately, I find that it makes many baked goods and breakfast cakes dark in color and tough in texture.

Making Your Own Baking Mixes

Most delicious g-free baked goods are made with a combination of three flours to mimic the texture and classic taste of the g-full version. Even when I have the energy to bake or the time to do so in my schedule, it always seems a lot of extra work to locate and measure out three different types of flours. So I prep the flour mixtures ahead of time; then I can just dig in when I'm ready to bake. In other words, one and done! Mix the Power Flours once per my directions below, and bake whenever you want!

You'll need to purchase four good-sized glass jars with pop-top latches and plastic gasket rings to keep your flour mixes fresh. Label the jars and store them in your g-free cupboard for up to five months. I am in the habit of mixing five batches at once because the jars I bought for this purpose hold that much mix, and because then I can have five Saturdays of waffles or pancakes or brownies ready to go!

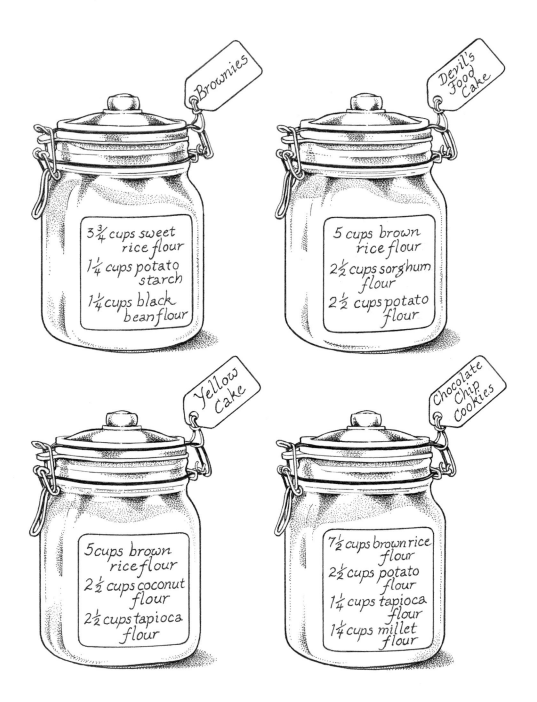

Brownies
(5 batches)

3¾ cups sweet white rice flour

1¼ cups potato starch

1¼ cups black bean flour

Devil's Food Cupcakes
(5 batches)

5 cups brown rice flour

2½ cups sweet sorghum flour

2½ cups potato flour

Yellow Birthday Cake or Classic Yellow Cupcakes
(5 batches)

5 cups brown rice flour

2½ cups coconut flour

2½ cups tapioca starch

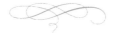

Chocolate Chip Cookies
(5 batches)

7½ cups brown rice flour

2½ cups potato flour

1¼ cups tapioca starch

1¼ cups millet flour

{Chapter 2}

Breakfasts to Remember

When first diagnosed with celiac disease, I thought traditional breakfast offerings would have to be a thing of my past, especially since my early experiments with gluten-free ingredients yielded heavy, gummy plates of pancakes and waffles. But times and available ingredients have changed, and so it's back to tender, buttery pancakes and crisp waffles . . . and happy mornings for us all. A bonus: I've developed combinations of multigrain flours for the best taste and texture, so you'll be getting more whole grains in your breakfast, too.

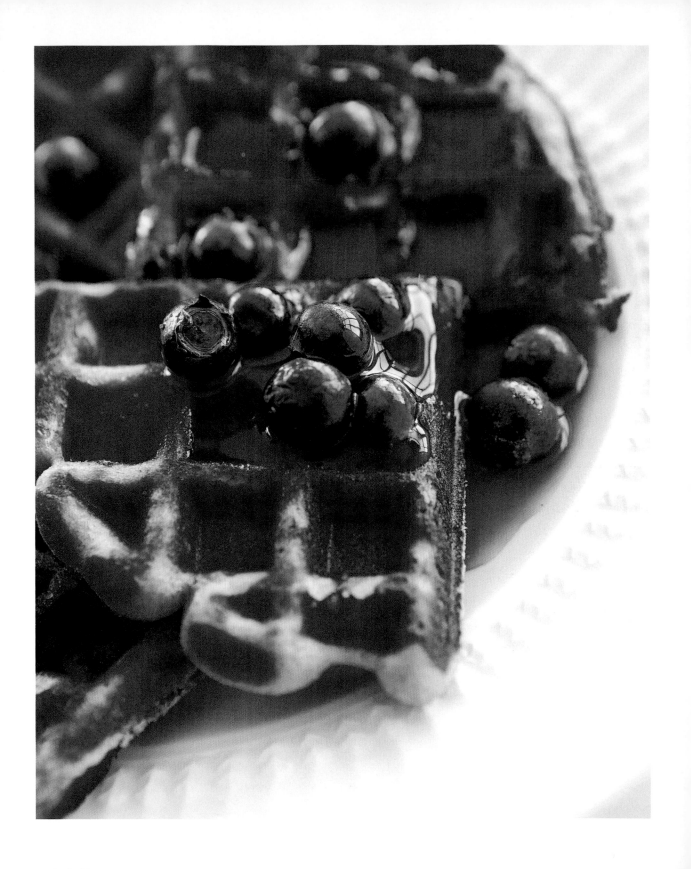

Blueberry Waffles

These crispy-on-the-outside, soft-on-the-inside waffles are naturally omega-3-fortified with high-fiber flax. Top them with a drizzle of maple syrup or additional blueberries for a fulfilling whole grain breakfast.

SERVES 6 (MAKES SIX 7-INCH WAFFLES)

4 eggs, separated
⅔ cup 2% milk
¼ cup gluten-free light sour cream
4 tablespoons (½ stick) salted butter, melted
Juice of 1 lemon
1 cup brown rice flour
¼ cup millet flour
¼ cup potato starch
¼ cup ground flax meal
2 tablespoons sugar
2 teaspoons baking powder
½ teaspoon baking soda
1 teaspoon guar gum
¼ teaspoon salt
1 cup fresh or frozen blueberries (defrosted if frozen)
Maple syrup, or blueberry or raspberry syrup (see page 29), for serving

1. Preheat a waffle maker according to the manufacturer's instructions.

2. Place the egg yolks, milk, sour cream, butter, and lemon juice in a large bowl. Whisk until well combined. Sprinkle the brown rice flour, millet flour, potato starch, flax meal, sugar, bak-

This is a great make-ahead-and-freeze recipe. The waffles are just as good warmed up in your g-free toaster days later!

ing powder, baking soda, and guar gum over the egg yolk mixture. Whisk until smooth.

3. Place the egg whites and salt in another large bowl. With an electric mixer on high speed, whisk the egg whites until stiff peaks form, about 2 minutes. Using a rubber spatula, fold a scoop of the egg whites into the batter; then carefully fold in the remaining whites with the rubber spatula.

4. Spoon ½ cup of the batter onto the waffle iron and cook according to the manufacturer's instructions. Keep the waffles warm while you repeat with the remaining batter. Serve hot, with the fresh or frozen berries and the syrup of your choice.

Elisabeth Hasselbeck

Pancakes with Homemade Berry Syrup

These light and fluffy pancakes will become a weekend tradition in your house. The main ingredient, sorghum, will give your breakfast a health boost: sorghum grains retain most of their nutrition, including a rich mix of antioxidants, because every part of the grain is ground for flour.

SERVES 4 (MAKES TWELVE 4-INCH PANCAKES)

Berry Syrup
1 pint fresh blueberries or raspberries
2 tablespoons powdered sugar
Grated zest of 1 lemon
1 tablespoon fresh lemon juice

Pancakes
4 tablespoons (½ stick) salted butter
1 cup sweet sorghum flour
½ cup sweet white rice flour
¼ cup tapioca starch
2 tablespoons granulated sugar
2½ teaspoons baking powder
1 teaspoon guar gum
¼ teaspoon salt
1½ cups 2% milk
2 eggs
½ teaspoon gluten-free vanilla extract

1. Make the berry syrup: Place the blueberries or raspberries in a small saucepan and add the powdered sugar, lemon zest, lemon juice, and ½ cup of water. Bring to a boil over high heat. Then reduce to a simmer and cook for 8 to 10 minutes, until the mixture becomes thick and the berries break apart. Set aside.

2. Melt the butter in a small saucepan over low heat, or microwave it in a glass bowl for 30 seconds on high power. Put aside to cool slightly.

3. In a large bowl, combine the sorghum flour, white rice flour, and tapioca starch, granulated sugar, baking powder, guar gum, and salt. Whisk until well blended.

4. Combine the milk, eggs, and vanilla in a small bowl, and stir with a fork until well blended. Pour the milk mixture and the melted butter into the flour mixture. Whisk until the flour mixture is well combined and a loose batter forms.

5. Heat a griddle over medium heat until hot. (To test if the griddle is hot enough, flick a drop of water onto it. It is ready if the drop dances quickly and evaporates.) Put half of the butter onto the griddle and spread it with a metal spatula. Drop the batter by ¼ cupfuls onto the griddle, spacing them about 3 inches apart. Cook until a few holes form on top of each pancake and the underside is golden brown, about 2 minutes. Carefully slide the metal spatula under each pancake and turn it over. Cook until the bottom is golden brown and the top is puffed, 1 to 2 minutes more. Using the spatula, transfer the pancakes to a serving plate. Repeat with the remaining butter and batter.

6. Serve the pancakes while still hot, with the berry syrup alongside.

The Deliciously Sophisticated Omelet

The Brie transforms this omelet into a grown-up version of a brunch classic. You're also starting out your day with a whole serving of vegetables, with the vitamin-C-rich broccoli. Double it up and refrigerate the extra egg mixture for a fast dinner, or for breakfast the next morning.

SERVES 4

Nonstick cooking spray
2 cups chopped broccoli florets
6 eggs, lightly beaten
¼ cup skim milk
¼ teaspoon salt
⅛ teaspoon freshly ground black pepper
1 tablespoon olive oil
¼ pound Brie cheese, cut into 6 slices

1. Heat a large skillet over high heat. Coat the skillet with cooking spray. Add the broccoli and cook for 1 minute, or until the broccoli starts to brown. Add ¼ cup of water and cover the skillet. Cook for 2 to 3 minutes more, until tender-crisp. Set aside.

2. Place the eggs, skim milk, salt, and pepper in a large bowl, and whisk gently to break up the yolks.

3. Heat another large skillet over high heat, and add the olive oil. Add the egg mixture and roll the skillet around until the eggs coat the inside. Reduce the heat to medium. Cook for about 1 minute, tilting the skillet and using a fork to pull the cooked egg into the center, until the egg mixture bunches like folds of fabric.

4. Reduce the heat to low and layer the cheese and broccoli on one side of the omelet. Flip the other side over on top of the fillings, and cover the skillet. Cook for 1 minute more to allow the cheese to melt and to warm the filling. Serve immediately.

Elisabeth Hasselbeck

Pumpkin Nut Quinoa Breakfast

Quinoa flakes deliver a creamy, satisfying breakfast porridge. Dress your bowl up with a swirl of vitamin-rich canned pumpkin, an ideal option for cool autumn mornings. Try cooking the quinoa in milk as well—this sweetens it and adds extra nutrition like vitamin D, calcium, and protein.

SERVES 4

¼ cup granulated sugar

½ teaspoon gluten-free ground cinnamon

1 teaspoon cornstarch

Pinch of salt

¼ teaspoon ground cloves

¼ teaspoon ground nutmeg

1 egg white

¼ teaspoon gluten-free vanilla extract

1 cup pecan halves

3½ cups water

1⅓ cups quinoa flakes

1 cup canned pumpkin

¼ cup half-and-half

¼ cup gluten-free light brown sugar

Quinoa is a tiny but mighty seed—a complete protein—grown in South America. It's high in manganese, which helps maintain blood sugar levels.

1. Preheat the oven to 300°F. Line a rimmed baking sheet with parchment paper.

2. Place the sugar, cinnamon, cornstarch, salt, ground cloves, and ground nutmeg in a plastic bag, seal the bag, and shake to mix.

3. Put the egg white and vanilla in a bowl, and beat until slightly foamy. Add the pecans and stir to coat them well. Using a slotted spoon, lift the pecans out of the bowl and transfer them to the bag of sugar and spices. Shake, making sure the pecans are well coated with the seasoning. Spread the pecans out on the prepared baking sheet, and bake for 30 minutes. Remove from the oven and let them cool on the baking sheet.

4. Meanwhile, place the water in a large saucepan and bring to a boil. Add the quinoa flakes and reduce the heat to medium. Cook for 10 to 15 minutes, until the liquid has decreased by half and the mixture is thick.

5. Combine the pumpkin and the half-and-half in a small bowl, and whisk until smooth. Swirl the pumpkin into the quinoa, and sprinkle with the brown sugar. Divide among four bowls, sprinkle with the chopped nuts, and serve immediately.

Frittata

This frittata is one of my family's go-to meals. It is the perfect way to use up bits of meat, sausage, cheese, and veggies/potatoes. It has also always been my main brunch recipe. Though it's easy to prep the same morning, I sometimes prep it at night with leftovers from dinner and let it sit in the fridge, then bake it fresh in the morning!

SERVES 4

10 eggs
¼ cup half-and-half
½ teaspoon salt
¼ teaspoon freshly ground black pepper
2 tablespoons olive oil
½ yellow onion, diced
½ green bell pepper, seeded and diced
1 cup canned black beans, drained and well rinsed
1 cup grated mozzarella or cheddar cheese

1. Preheat the oven to 350°F.

2. Place the eggs, half-and-half, salt, and pepper in a large bowl. Whisk to combine, and set aside.

3. Heat an 8-inch ovenproof skillet with high sides over medium-high heat. Add 1 tablespoon of the olive oil, the onion, and the green pepper. Cook, stirring occasionally, until tender, 3 to 4 minutes. Transfer to a small bowl.

4. In the same skillet over medium-low heat, warm the remaining 1 tablespoon olive oil. Add the egg mixture and cook for 1 minute, until the edges start to bubble. Using a metal spoon, pull the cooked egg edges toward the center of the pan, allowing the raw egg to run to the edges of the skillet.

5. Scatter the cooked vegetables, the beans, and the cheese over the eggs. Transfer the skillet to the oven and bake for 10 to 12 minutes or until the frittata is firm in the middle and does not jiggle when you shake the skillet. Remove the skillet from the oven and let it cool for 5 minutes.

6. To loosen the frittata, run a paring knife around the edges, between the frittata and the skillet. Gently shake the pan to loosen the frittata, sliding a spatula underneath to loosen it further. Slide it onto a serving plate, and cut it into 8 equal wedges. Serve immediately, or cool completely before storing in an airtight container in the refrigerator for up to 3 days. Reheat for 20 minutes in a 200°F oven.

Fried Egg Sandwich with Chipotle Mayo

What a way to wake up! Toasting the bagel in the skillet with a smear of butter keeps it moist, and the chipotle mayo (which can be made ahead of time) adds a flavor punch. Top the sandwich with baby spinach to boost the vitamin content or with a piece of fresh romaine lettuce to add vitamin A. Once you bite into this, you will be ready to tackle whatever comes your way!

SERVES 2

¼ cup gluten-free light mayonnaise

1 tablespoon adobo sauce from a can of gluten-free chipotle en adobo

Juice and grated zest of 1 lime

1 garlic clove, minced

¼ teaspoon granulated sugar

4 slices gluten-free bread; or 2 gluten-free bagels, cut in half

4 teaspoons salted butter

Nonstick cooking spray

2 eggs

⅛ teaspoon freshly ground black pepper

2 slices white cheese, such as cheddar or Muenster

2 slices romaine lettuce leaves, or a handful of baby spinach leaves

2 slices tomato

> *My husband, Tim, loves it when I make these for his morning commute to work. Confession: Truthfully, though I wish I could, I don't make them all the time. I think the true sign of their deliciousness is that he wishes I made them more often!*

   1. Place the mayonnaise, adobo sauce, lime juice and zest, garlic, and sugar in a small bowl. Stir well to combine, and set aside.

   2. Heat a large skillet over medium heat. Spread each bread slice, or the inside of each bagel slice, with 1 teaspoon of the butter. Place the bread or bagels, butter side down, in the skillet. Cook for 1 to 2 minutes, pressing down on them with a small heavy saucepan or with the underside of a metal spatula. When the bread or bagels have browned, set them aside.

3. Remove pan from heat and coat the same skillet with a thick layer of cooking spray. Carefully crack both eggs into the skillet, and sprinkle with the pepper. Cook for 2 to 3 minutes, until the edges of the eggs start to brown. Cover the skillet, and cook for another 2 to 3 minutes, until the whites are completely cooked through but the yolks are still soft. Place a slice of cheese over each egg during the last minute of cooking.

4. Transfer each fried egg to a slice of toast or a bagel half. Top with the lettuce or spinach and the tomato slices, and cover with the remaining toast or bagel halves.

Elisabeth Hasselbeck

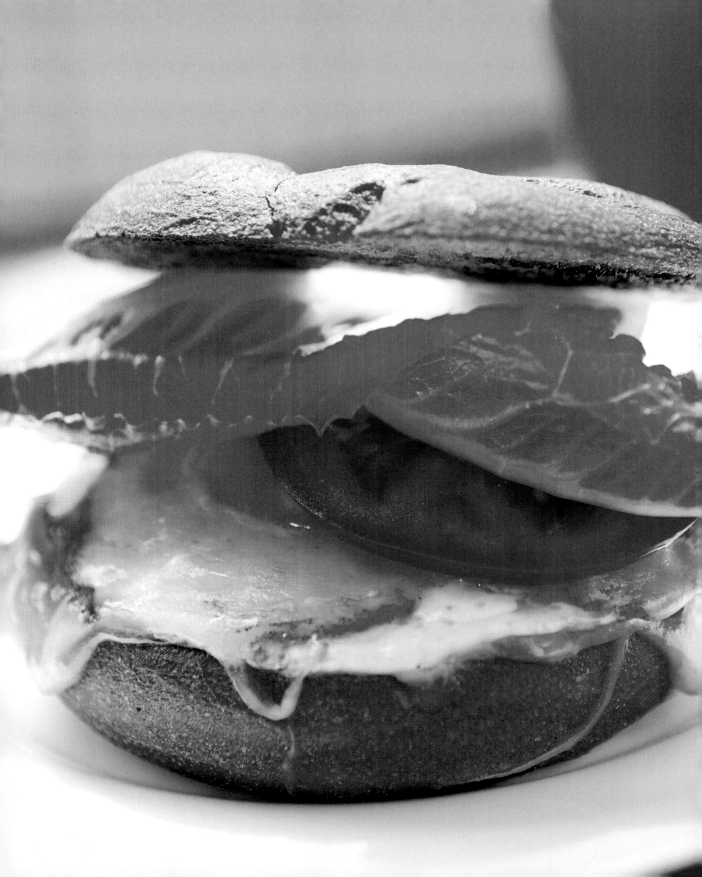

Fruit Salad with Dreamy Whipped Topping

This fast, no-cook recipe will make a colorful addition to your next potluck or summer cookout. With the whipped topping, this fruit salad becomes an indulgent treat that is still healthy enough for breakfast but can also be served for dessert.

SERVES 4

1 cup plain 2% Greek yogurt
½ cup gluten-free light sour cream
3 tablespoons powdered sugar
1 teaspoon grated orange or lemon zest
1 cup cubed cantaloupe
1 cup cubed honeydew
1 cup blueberries
1 cup raspberries
1 cup red, black, or green seedless grapes, cut in half
¼ cup packed fresh mint leaves

1. Prepare the whipped topping: Place the yogurt, sour cream, powdered sugar, and orange or lemon zest in a large bowl. Whisk until smooth. Cover and refrigerate until ready to use. The topping will keep for 1 day, refrigerated.

2. Place the cantaloupe, honeydew, blueberries, raspberries, grapes, and mint in a large bowl. Toss to combine.

3. Spoon the fruit into four small bowls, and add a spoonful of the whipped topping to each one.

Elisabeth Hasselbeck

French Toast with Caramel Rum Bananas

The rum-scented banana topping gives this French toast gourmet flair. To make it kid-friendly, hold the rum and instead dust the French toast with powdered sugar (which we call "snow" in our house), then top it with freshly sliced strawberries or syrup.

SERVES 4

4 eggs
1 cup 2% milk
4 tablespoons firmly packed gluten-free dark brown sugar
1 teaspoon gluten-free ground cinnamon
Pinch of salt
8 slices gluten-free sandwich bread
Nonstick canola oil spray
2 tablespoons salted butter
4 ripe bananas, cut into ½-inch-thick slices
½ cup gluten-free dark rum
1 teaspoon gluten-free vanilla extract, or ½ teaspoon vanilla powder
1 teaspoon gluten-free almond extract or hazelnut extract (optional)

G-free breads absorb and hold moisture well, making them the ideal vehicle for eggs, cinnamon, and milk.

1. Preheat the oven to 200°F.

2. In a large shallow bowl, whisk together the eggs, milk, 2 tablespoons of the brown sugar, the cinnamon, and the salt until well combined. Poke the bread with the tines of a fork. Pour the egg mixture into a deep pie dish. Soak 1 bread slice, turning it over once, for 1 to 2 minutes in the egg mixture. Transfer the soaked bread to a plate, and repeat with the remaining bread and egg mixture.

3. Heat two large skillets over medium-high heat. Remove skillets from heat and coat the inside of both skillets with a thick layer of cooking spray. Add 4 bread slices to each skillet and cook, turning them over once, until golden, 2 to 3 minutes per side. Transfer to the oven to keep warm.

4. Heat a small skillet over high heat. Add the butter, bananas, and remaining 2 tablespoons brown sugar. Cook for about 1 minute, until the bananas start to brown. Off the heat, add the rum, vanilla extract or powder, almond or hazelnut extract if using, and 1 tablespoon of water. Place the skillet over low heat and cook for 2 to 3 minutes, until a thick sauce forms.

5. Serve the French toast immediately, topped with the banana sauce.

Blueberry Muffins

Visiting a friend or having a bake sale? These are perfect in a gift basket with some homemade flavored butter: Mash ¼ teaspoon gluten-free ground cinnamon into 4 tablespoons of room-temperature salted butter.

MAKES 12 MUFFINS

1 cup sweet sorghum flour

½ cup millet flour

½ cup tapioca starch

1 cup granulated sugar

2 teaspoons baking powder

¼ teaspoon baking soda

⅛ teaspoon salt

1 teaspoon guar gum

1 cup blueberries

1 cup 2% milk

8 tablespoons (1 stick) salted butter, at room temperature

2 eggs

1 teaspoon gluten-free vanilla extract or powder

6 teaspoons Sugar in the Raw or brown turbinado sugar

You can always spot gluten-free spices because they tend to clump. No problem: they taste just as good, clumps and all!

1. Preheat the oven to 400°F. Line a 12-cup muffin tin with paper muffin liners.

2. In a bowl, stir together the three types of flour, granulated sugar, baking powder, baking soda, salt, and guar gum. Add the berries and stir just until they are coated with flour (this will keep the berries from bursting and turning the wet batter blue). Set aside.

3. In another bowl, whisk together the milk, butter, eggs, and vanilla extract or powder until smooth. Add the flour mixture and stir just until blended, about 10 turns with a wooden spoon. Spoon the batter into the prepared muffin cups, filling each one to the top of the paper liner. Sprinkle ½ teaspoon of the raw sugar over each muffin. Bake until the tops of the muffins spring back to the touch, 18 to 20 minutes.

4. Transfer the muffin tin to a wire rack and let it cool for 5 minutes. Then remove the muffins from the tin. Store the muffins in an airtight container on the counter for up to 3 days.

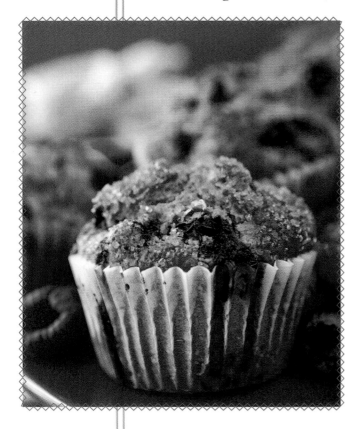

Elisabeth Hasselbeck

Coconut Raspberry Muffins

I've always loved the flavor combo of raspberry and coconut. These muffins are wonderfully rich in taste and surprisingly interesting on the palate.

MAKES 12 MUFFINS

½ cup sweet sorghum flour

¼ cup brown rice flour

¼ cup potato flour

2 teaspoons baking powder

2 teaspoons guar gum

¼ teaspoon baking soda

⅛ teaspoon salt

⅔ cup granulated sugar

4 tablespoon (½ stick) salted butter, melted

2 eggs

1 cup 2% milk

1 cup gluten-free sweetened shredded coconut

1 cup fresh or defrosted frozen raspberries

6 teaspoons Sugar in the Raw or brown turbinado sugar

1. Preheat the oven to 400°F. Line a 12-cup muffin tin with paper muffin liners.

2. In a bowl, stir together the three types of flour, baking powder, guar gum, baking soda, and salt. Set aside.

3. Place the granulated sugar and the butter in a large bowl and whisk until well combined. Whisk in the eggs, one at a time, until well combined. Then whisk in the milk. Add the flour mixture and stir just until blended, about 8 turns with a wooden spoon. Add the coconut and raspberries and stir just until evenly incorporated.

4. Spoon the batter into the prepared muffin cups, filling each one about three-fourths full. Sprinkle the raw sugar over the muffin tops. Bake until the muffins are firm to the touch in the center, 20 to 22 minutes.

5. Transfer the muffin tin to a wire rack and let it cool for 5 minutes. Then remove the muffins from the tin. Store the muffins in an airtight container on the counter for up to 4 days.

Elisabeth Hasselbeck

Egg Muffins

These beauties are the ultimate family-pleaser. My kids call them "egg cupcakes" and love them because I let them eat the muffins with their hands. I love them because they give everyone a protein-rich and colorful start to the day.

Try this: Let your kids or guests toss ingredients they like into each muffin cup before you add the eggs. For large groups, I set out some options in small glass prep bowls: sliced pepperoni, cooked turkey bacon, chopped scallions, salsa, black beans, feta cheese, olives, and fresh herbs make endless combinations.

MAKES 12 MUFFINS

12 eggs
½ teaspoon baking powder
¼ teaspoon salt
¼ teaspoon freshly ground black pepper
2 cups grated cheddar cheese
3 scallions, finely chopped, using both white and green parts
½ red bell pepper, seeded and chopped
5 ounces mushrooms, thinly sliced
1 cup diced gluten-free Canadian bacon or deli ham; or 4 slices cooked pork bacon, chopped

This recipe is easy to cut in half—and/or the muffins freeze well if you make the whole batch.

1. Preheat the oven to 375°F. Coat a 12-cup muffin tin with nonstick spray.

2. Place the eggs in a large bowl and add the baking powder, salt, and black pepper. Whisk well to combine.

3. In the bottom of the prepared muffin cups, layer the cheese, scallions, red bell pepper, mushrooms, and Canadian bacon, ham, or pork bacon. Pour the egg mixture into the muffin cups, filling each one three-fourths full.

4. Bake for 15 to 20 minutes, until the egg muffins rise and the edges are slightly browned. Serve immediately.

Baked egg muffins can be frozen and reheated: Let the cooked muffins cool completely. Then wrap each egg muffin in a piece of wax paper, transfer them to a large zipper-lock bag, and freeze for up to 1 month. To reheat, preheat the oven to 200°F. Warm the muffins for 10 minutes or until they are warmed through. Serve immediately.

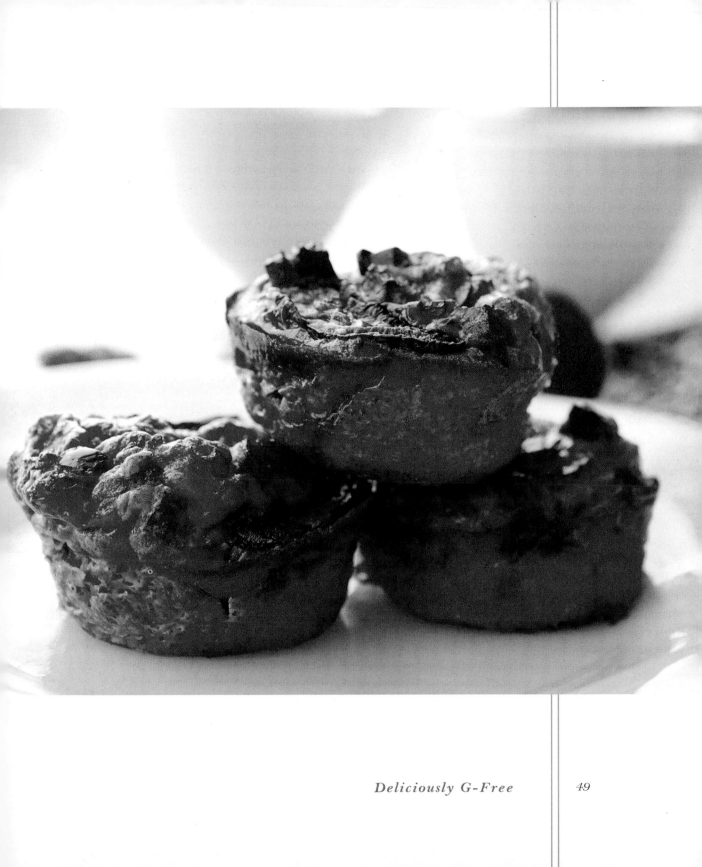

{Chapter 3}

All-Star Appetizers

In my early days of eating and cooking g-free, I never really tried to *entertain* with my g-free food. I usually just made all my dishes with full-on gluten and then didn't eat them—I didn't want my guests to have to eat food that was less flavorful or less delicious than they were used to enjoying at our house. But in testing recipes for this book (and for my life!), I've become a g-free gourmet, and now when I entertain, I serve food that *no one would believe is g-free* if I didn't announce the fact. Whether you're throwing a lavish party, preparing a picnic, or feeding a crowd around the television at game time, these recipes will make your food the star of the show. Welcome back to flavor and variety!

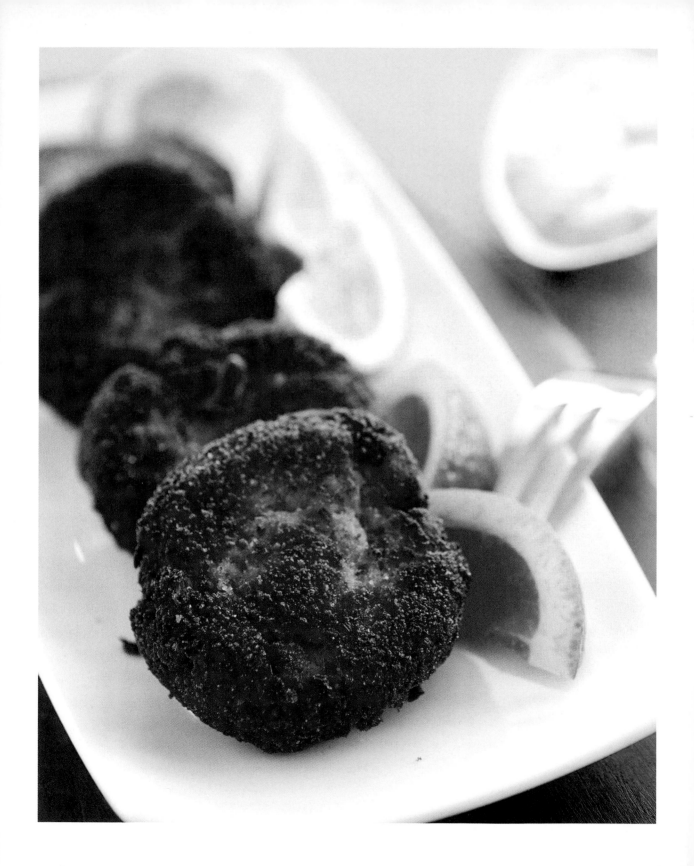

Crab Cakes with Homemade Tartar Sauce

Fresh bread crumbs make a super-crisp, uniform coating that can be seasoned with any herb or spice you like. To make them, simply tear up gluten-free bread and pulse the pieces in a food processor until small, fluffy crumbs form.

SERVES 4 (MAKES 4 LARGE OR 8 APPETIZER-SIZE CRAB CAKES)

Tartar Sauce
1 cup gluten-free light mayonnaise
½ cup gluten-free sweet pickle relish
Grated zest and juice of 1 lemon

Crabcakes
2 scallions thinly sliced, using both white and green parts
2 tablespoons chopped fresh flat-leaf parsley
2 teaspoons gluten-free Dijon mustard
½ teaspoon salt
¼ teaspoon freshly ground white or black pepper
¼ teaspoon ground cayenne pepper
¾ pound lump crabmeat
2 cups fresh gluten-free bread crumbs
2 tablespoons olive oil
¼ cup chopped fresh chives
1 lemon, cut into wedges

Four slices of g-free bread will yield about 2 cups of bread crumbs.

1. Prepare the tartar sauce: Place ½ cup of the mayonnaise in a small bowl, and add the pickle relish and the lemon zest. Stir well to combine. Cover and refrigerate until ready to serve.

2. In a large bowl, combine the lemon juice with the remaining ½ cup mayonnaise and the scallions, parsley, mustard, salt, pepper, and cayenne. Stir to combine. Add the crabmeat and 1 cup of the bread crumbs. Using a spatula, gently fold all the ingredients together until the mixture comes together in a sticky but firm mass.

3. Shape the crab mixture into 8 small patties. Spread the remaining 1 cup bread crumbs out on a plate or a piece of wax paper. Coat the patties in the bread crumbs and place them on another piece of wax paper. Chill for at least 1 hour before cooking.

4. Preheat the oven to 350°F.

5. Heat a large ovenproof skillet over medium-high heat and add the olive oil. Cook the patties until golden brown on both sides, 3 to 4 minutes total. (Reduce the heat if the bread-crumb coating begins to brown too quickly.) Slide the skillet into the oven and bake for 10 to 15 minutes, to warm the center of the cakes.

6. Sprinkle the chives over the crab cakes and serve warm, with the tartar sauce and lemon wedges alongside.

Kale Chips

My kids dug into these the first time I made them: what a delicious surprise! These are a great snack for movie night and a healthy pre-dinner munchie to tide the gang (and you) over while you cook.

SERVES 4

1 large bunch kale (about 1 pound)
2 tablespoons olive oil
¼ teaspoon salt

1. Preheat the oven to 400°F.

2. Trim off and discard the tough stems of the kale and rinse the leaves under cold running water. Wrap the leaves tightly in a dish towel to dry them.

3. Place the olive oil in a large bowl. Unwrap the kale leaves and coarsely chop them. Add them to the bowl and toss them in the oil, rubbing them to coat them well. Sprinkle with the salt.

4. Divide the kale between two ungreased baking sheets and bake for 8 to 10 minutes, until the leaves are crisp. Serve immediately.

Looking to recharge your battery? High-voltage kale will give you a lift, providing nearly 100 percent of your daily needs for vitamins K, A, and C in just 1 cup.

Pork Pot Stickers

I thought I had dumped dumplings for good, until I figured this one out! Soft, tender Chinese dumplings are not a "no-no" any longer! Even if you don't have a pasta maker, making this fresh pasta dough is fast and easy; it rolls out easily with a wooden rolling pin or even a coffee mug.

MAKES 24 POT STICKERS

This dough works equally well stuffed with ricotta cheese for ravioli.

Dough
½ cup tapioca starch
½ cup potato flour
2 tablespoons cornstarch
½ teaspoon salt
2 teaspoons xanthan gum
2 large eggs, lightly beaten
2 egg yolks
2 tablespoons olive oil

Filling
1 tablespoon Asian sesame oil
2 cups finely chopped napa cabbage
¼ pound ground pork
2 carrots finely diced
1 cup thinly sliced shiitake mushrooms
1 garlic clove, minced
1 teaspoon minced peeled fresh ginger
2 tablespoons gluten-free soy sauce
1 tablespoon fish sauce

Elisabeth Hasselbeck

1. Make the dough: In a medium bowl, combine the tapioca starch, potato flour, cornstarch, salt, and xanthan gum. Make a well in the center and add the eggs, egg yolks, and olive oil. Stir until all the flour is combined.

2. Work the dough into a firm ball with your fingers, and knead it for about 1 minute, until the surface of the dough is smooth. Cut the dough into 24 equal pieces and roll them into balls. Cover with a dish towel and set aside.

3. Prepare the filling: Heat a large skillet over high heat. Add the sesame oil, cabbage, pork, carrots, mushrooms, garlic, ginger, soy sauce, and fish sauce. Cook, stirring often, until the cabbage starts to soften and the pork is cooked, 4 to 5 minutes. Set aside.

4. Place 1 cup of cold water in a small bowl. Lightly flour the countertop (a pinch or two of tapioca starch will do it). Using a rolling pin, roll out each dough ball into a 4-inch disk, and place them on a baking sheet. Cover the disks with a towel to keep them from drying out. To fill the dumplings, place a tablespoon of the filling in the center of each disk. Dip your finger in the water and run it along the edge of the disk. Fold the dough over to make a half-moon shape, and press the edges closed with your fingers. Return the filled dumplings to the baking sheet and cover with the towel.

5. Fill a large stockpot with water and bring it to a boil. Add about 10 dumplings and cook for 2 to 3 minutes, until the dough is soft; remove with a slotted spoon. Repeat with the remaining dumplings, and serve immediately.

Swedish Meatballs

These dinner party/Sunday football game staples are so good that I recommend making a double batch so you can avoid the "why aren't there any more meatballs?" look. For fun, I often create meatball "drumsticks" for the kids, making it easy to dip the meatballs (and to eat with their hands): Simply skewer several meatballs onto lollipop sticks from the craft store, or onto bamboo skewers (cut off the sharp ends to avoid boo-boos).

SERVES 8 (MAKES 36 MEATBALLS)

This finger-friendly food is the perfect nosh for a cocktail party or a girls' night in.

1 tablespoon salted butter
½ medium onion, finely chopped
2¼ teaspoons salt
½ pound ground pork
½ pound ground turkey
½ cup millet flour
1 large egg
½ teaspoon gluten-free ground allspice
½ teaspoon gluten-free mustard powder
½ teaspoon freshly ground black pepper
3 tablespoons canola oil
4 celery stalks, thinly sliced on the diagonal
½ cup orange marmalade
¼ cup gluten-free beef broth

1. Melt the butter in a medium skillet over medium-high heat. Add the onion and ¼ teaspoon of the salt, and cook until golden brown, 4 to 6 minutes. Transfer to a large bowl.

Elisabeth Hasselbeck

2. Add the ground pork, ground turkey, millet flour, egg, ground allspice, mustard powder, and ground pepper to the large bowl. Mix gently with your hands until combined.

3. Dampen your hands, and form the mixture into 36 small meatballs, about 1 tablespoon each. Put them on a parchment paper–lined baking sheet, cover it with plastic wrap, and refrigerate for at least 4 hours or overnight.

4. Heat the canola oil in a large skillet over medium-high heat. Cook the meatballs in batches, turning them occasionally, until all sides are lightly browned, 3 to 4 minutes. Skewer each meatball with a toothpick along with a slice of the celery.

5. Make the dipping sauce: Place the marmalade and beef broth in a small saucepan and bring to a simmer over medium-low heat. Cook 2 to 3 minutes, stirring often until a thick sauce forms. Serve immediately with the meatball skewers.

Crostini Platter

Crostini make a great party food that covers all the bases. These have classic Italian flavors that everyone loves and that are also appropriate for vegetarians.

SERVES 8

For the BLT option, substitute ½ pound gluten-free cooked bacon for the mozzarella. Use 2 cups of baby arugula, chopped, and sprinkle over crostini in place of the balsamic vinegar.

1 cup gluten-free balsamic vinegar
8 slices gluten-free bread, cut in half diagonally; or 8 1-inch-thick slices gluten-free baguette
4 vine-ripened tomatoes (about 1 pound total), diced
½ cup fresh basil leaves, torn or thinly sliced
2 tablespoons finely minced red onion (optional)
2 tablespoons olive oil
¼ teaspoon salt
⅛ teaspoon coarsely ground black pepper
1 pound fresh mozzarella cheese, cubed or sliced

1. Preheat the oven to 350°F.

2. Place the balsamic vinegar in a small saucepan. Bring to a simmer and cook for 15 to 20 minutes, until it has reduced by half. Set aside.

3. Meanwhile, place the bread slices on a baking sheet and bake until crisp and golden, 15 to 18 minutes. Set aside.

4. Place the tomatoes, ¼ cup of the basil, the onion if using, and the olive oil, salt, and pepper in a large bowl. Toss to combine.

5. To assemble the crostini, lay a piece of mozzarella on each piece of toasted bread and spoon 2 tablespoons of the tomato mixture on top. Transfer the crostini to a platter, and drizzle with the balsamic syrup and top with the remaining basil. Serve immediately.

Elisabeth Hasselbeck

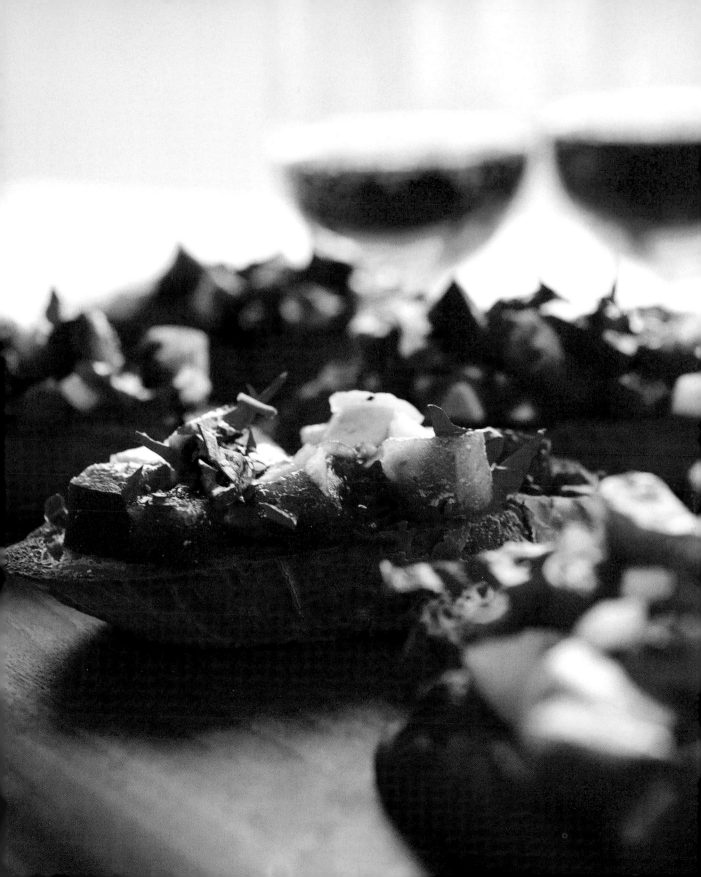

Tri-Color Melon and Prosciutto

The ingredients in this recipe are classic antipasto offerings from my family table, only this time . . . served on sticks! With no silverware required, this is a great poolside treat or rooftop appetizer. For an elegant patio or rooftop dinner, serve these as a first course with a glass of chilled white wine, such as a Sauvignon Blanc or Sancerre.

MAKES ABOUT 30 PIECES

1 large cantaloupe or honeydew melon; you can also use Ambrosia melon
    or Santa Claus melon or some combination of any of them as you like
Juice of 1 lemon
¼ pound thinly sliced imported prosciutto di Parma
1 8-ounce container of fresh cherry-size mozzarella cheese balls, each ball
    cut in half
1 cup fresh basil leaves
½ cup extra-virgin olive oil
¼ teaspoon salt

1. Cut the melon in half and remove the seeds. Using a melon baller, scoop the melon flesh into small balls. Place the melon balls in a bowl and sprinkle the lemon juice all over them.

2. Cut the prosciutto into narrow strips, and wrap each strip around a melon ball. Pierce through the prosciutto and melon with a toothpick, and spear a piece of mozzarella as well. Arrange the skewers on a platter.

3. Place the basil, olive oil, and salt in a blender or mini-chopper, and blend until the basil leaves are chopped. Strain the basil mixture over a small bowl. Drizzle the basil oil over the skewers and serve immediately.

Elisabeth Hasselbeck

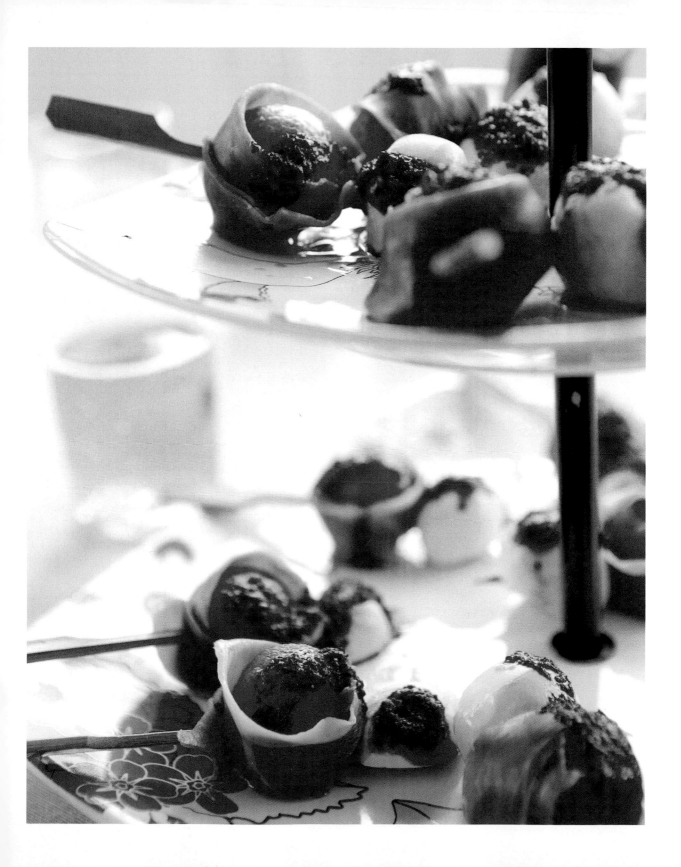

Potato Skins with Cheddar, Chives, and Bacon

Game time food is a must in my house. Serve these alongside the Chili Cheese Fries (page 68) and a big bowl of creamy guacamole (page 76) for a snacking extravaganza that screams "victory!"

SERVES 8

Restaurant versions of this fan favorite tend to be dripping with fat and loaded with calories. Using cooking spray and scaling back on the cheese lightens up the fat without losing flavor.

8 small Idaho potatoes (about 2½ pounds total), scrubbed and dried
Nonstick cooking spray
4 slices gluten-free bacon (about 3 ounces), finely diced
1 teaspoon gluten-free mild chili powder
¼ teaspoon salt
½ pound broccoli florets, coarsely chopped (about 4 cups)
½ cup pickled jalapeños, chopped
1 cup grated cheddar cheese (about ¼ pound)
2 scallions, thinly sliced, using both white and green parts

1. Preheat the oven to 450°F. Line a plate with paper towels and set it aside.

2. Pierce the potatoes in several places with a fork and wrap each one in aluminum foil. Bake for 50 minutes to 1 hour, until soft to the touch.

3. Meanwhile, coat a small skillet with cooking spray. Add the bacon and cook over medium heat, stirring occasionally, until golden brown. Transfer to the paper towel–lined plate to drain.

4. When the potatoes are ready, unwrap them and set them aside for 5 minutes or until they are cool enough to handle. Then cut the potatoes into quarters and allow them to cool for another

Elisabeth Hasselbeck

5 minutes. Using a spoon, carefully scoop out the flesh, leaving a ⅛-inch-thick shell intact. Reserve the scooped-out potato flesh for another use.

5. Coat both the inside and the outside of the potato shells with cooking spray, and sprinkle with the chili powder and salt. Place the potatoes, skin side down, on a baking sheet and bake until the skins are crisp and the edges are golden brown, about 20 minutes.

6. In the meantime, prepare the filling: Bring water to a simmer in the bottom of a vegetable steamer, place the broccoli in the steamer basket, cover, and steam until it is crisp-tender, 3 to 4 minutes. Set aside.

7. Sprinkle the broccoli, bacon, and jalapeños onto the potato skins. Sprinkle with the cheese. Reduce the oven temperature to 400°F, return the potatoes to the oven, and bake until the cheese has melted, about 5 minutes. Top with the scallions.

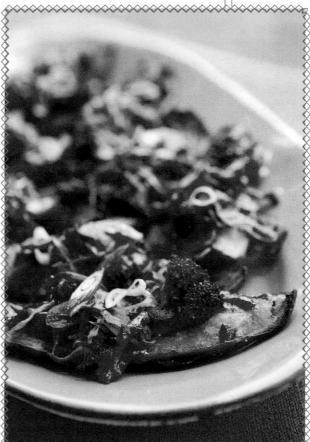

Stuffed Mushrooms

A classic starter for any holiday meal, these mushrooms travel well. You can bake them hours ahead of time, cover them, and then warm them for 10 minutes in a 200°F oven before serving.

SERVES 8

2 10-ounce packages large white mushrooms
1 tablespoon olive oil
2 gluten-free Italian sausage links, mild or hot, removed from casing
½ red or yellow onion, finely chopped
2 garlic cloves, minced
¼ cup chopped flat-leaf parsley
½ teaspoon salt
¼ teaspoon freshly ground black pepper
¼ teaspoon gluten-free red pepper flakes (optional)
½ cup freshly grated Pecorino Romano cheese
¼ cup fresh goat cheese
¼ cup 2% milk

1. Preheat the oven to 400°F.

2. Remove the stems from the mushrooms. Chop half of the stems (discard the remaining stems or save them for another recipe). Heat a large skillet over high heat. Add the olive oil, the chopped mushroom stems, and the sausage, onion, garlic, parsley, salt, black pepper, and red pepper flakes if using. Reduce the heat to medium and cook, stirring occasionally and breaking up the sausage with the back of a spoon, until the sausage is cooked through and no longer pink, 7 to 9 minutes. Remove the skillet from the heat and add ¼ cup of the Pecorino, the goat cheese, and the milk. Stir gently for 1 minute or until the cheeses melt.

Elisabeth Hasselbeck

3. Arrange the mushroom caps snugly in an 8-inch square baking dish, cap side down. Stuff each mushroom with a heaping tablespoon of the sausage stuffing and sprinkle them with the remaining Pecorino.

4. Bake for 10 to 15 minutes, until the stuffing is browned and the mushroom caps are soft. Transfer to a platter and serve immediately.

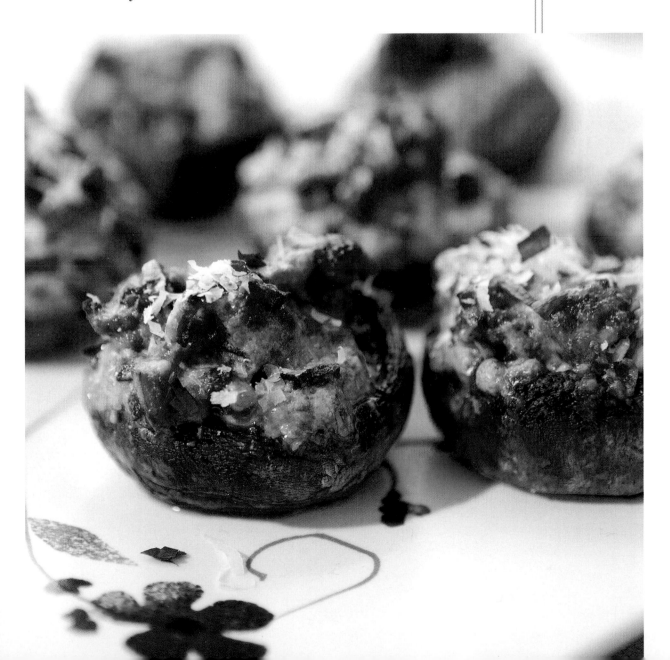

Chili Cheese Fries

Bring the bar food to your home! This hearty snack is great for a game, guys' night in, or last-minute appetizer.

SERVES 8

There are many healthy, tasty frozen g-free fries on the market. Keep a couple of bags in your freezer along with some ground beef, and you'll be in good shape to serve surprise drop-in guests.

1 16-ounce bag frozen gluten-free wedge-cut potato fries

1 cup gluten-free beef broth

½ teaspoon cornstarch

1 tablespoon olive oil

1 red or green bell pepper, seeded and chopped

½ red onion, minced

2 garlic cloves, minced

¼ teaspoon salt

½ pound lean ground beef

1 tablespoon gluten-free mild chili powder

½ teaspoon gluten-free ground cumin

1 15-ounce can kidney beans, drained and well rinsed

2 cups shredded cheddar cheese

1. Preheat the oven to 400°F.

2. Divide the frozen fries between two baking sheets, and bake them for 20 to 25 minutes or according to the package instructions.

3. While the fries are baking, place the beef broth and cornstarch in a small bowl, and whisk until smooth. Set aside.

4. Heat a large skillet over high heat and add the olive oil. Add the bell pepper, onion, garlic, and salt. Cook, stirring often, until the pepper softens, 3 to 4 minutes. Add the beef and cook for 1 to 2 minutes without stirring so it can brown. Sprinkle the chili powder and cumin over the beef. Continue to cook for 1 minute more, breaking up the beef with the back of a spoon. Add the beans and the cornstarch mixture, and reduce the heat to low. Simmer for 15 to 20 minutes, until the mixture is thick.

5. When the fries are crisp, transfer them to an 8 × 12-inch casserole. Spoon the chili over the fries and sprinkle with the cheese. Transfer the casserole to the oven and bake for 5 to 10 minutes, until the cheese is bubbling and the chili is hot. Serve immediately.

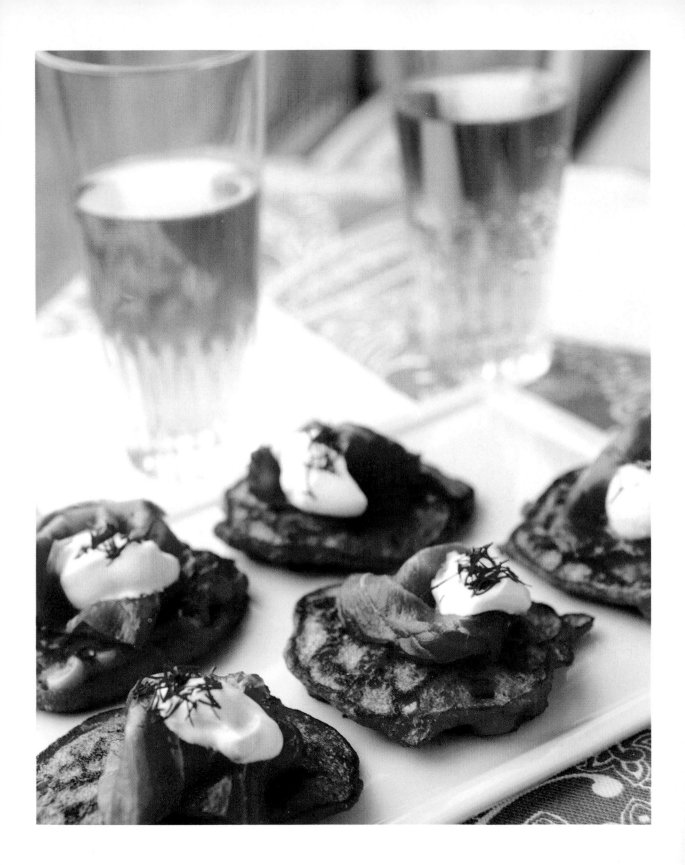

Smoked Salmon on Corn Fritters

Use this as an elegant start to a dinner party or as a new dish for your brunch recipe collection. Look for wild smoked salmon to get your dose of omega-3's; farm-raised salmon does not contain this valuable antioxidant.

SERVES 4

1 cup frozen or fresh corn kernels (from about 2 large ears)
¼ cup finely ground gluten-free cornmeal
¼ cup brown rice flour
2 tablespoons tapioca starch
1 teaspoon baking powder
¼ teaspoon salt
¼ teaspoon gluten-free mild or hot chili powder
¼ teaspoon freshly ground black pepper
1 large jalapeño, seeded and chopped
½ cup 2% milk
2 tablespoons salted butter, melted and cooled
1 egg, lightly beaten
Nonstick cooking spray
16 small slices smoked salmon
1 cup crème fraîche or sour cream
1 tablespoon fresh dill, chopped

These fritters can be made up to 1 hour ahead. Transfer them to a wire rack to cool; then keep them on a covered plate before serving at room temperature, or rewarm them in a toaster oven before serving.

1. If using frozen corn, rinse it under hot running water for 1 minute to defrost it. Drain well.

2. In a large bowl, whisk together the cornmeal, brown rice flour, tapioca starch, baking powder, salt, chili powder, and black pepper.

3. Make a well in the center of the cornmeal mixture, and add the corn, jalapeño, milk, butter, and egg. Starting from the center, mix the wet ingredients with a wooden spoon, slowly combining them with the cornmeal mixture until it is just combined, about 10 turns of the spoon. Set aside for 10 minutes.

4. Place a large griddle or skillet over medium-high heat. When it is hot, carefully coat it with cooking spray. Using a half-filled ¼ cup measure, pour the batter onto the hot griddle and spread it out to form fritters about 4 inches in diameter. Cook until they are golden on the bottom and bubbles are starting to appear on the surface, about 3 minutes. Then turn them over and cook until the other side is golden and the center is set, about 2 minutes more. Transfer the fritters to a plate and keep them warm while you cook the remainder (you should have 8 total).

5. Set out four plates. Place 2 fritters on each plate and top each with two slices of smoked salmon, a spoonful of crème fraîche or sour cream, and a garnish of chopped fresh dill. Serve immediately.

Elisabeth Hasselbeck

Buffalo Chicken Tenders

If you can't get enough wings but have had enough of the fried and heavily caloric version, you and your guests will be more than happy with this healthy yet spicy makeover. Even a wing connoisseur will love these tenders and figure them for the "real deal."

SERVES 4

¼ cup hot sauce
1 teaspoon gluten-free hot paprika
¼ teaspoon salt
1 pound chicken tenders
1 tablespoon salted butter

A quarter pound of these tenders has only 144 calories and 4 grams of fat, with all the spicy kick of the classic version you may be used to.

1. Preheat the oven to 375°F.

2. Combine the hot sauce, paprika, and salt in a small bowl. Brush this marinade over all surfaces of the chicken.

3. Grease an 11 × 7-inch baking dish with the butter, and spread the chicken out in the dish. Cover, and marinate in the refrigerator for 30 minutes.

4. Bake, uncovered, for about 15 minutes or until the chicken is no longer pink in the center.

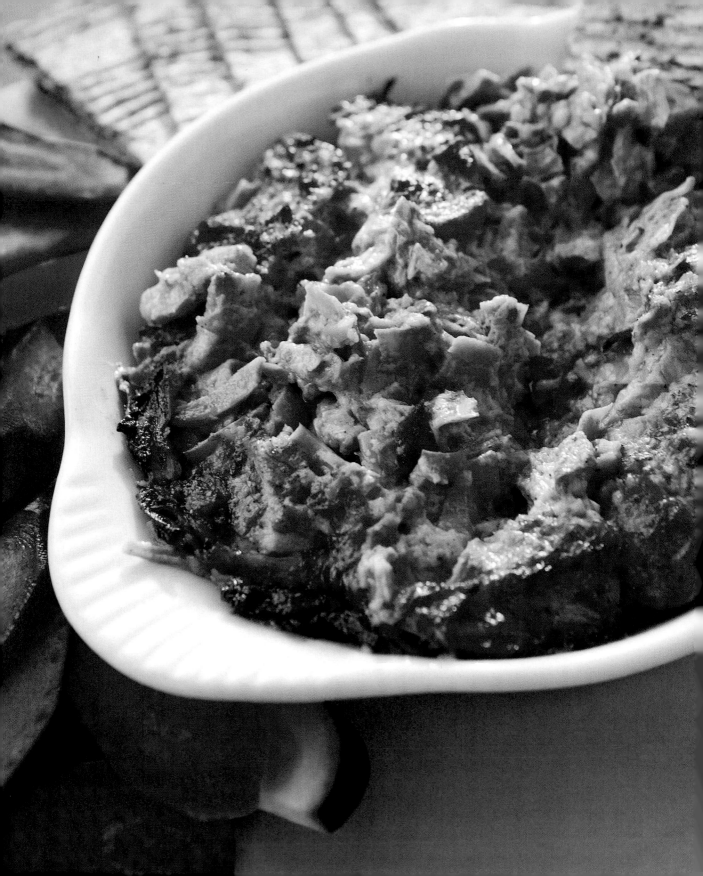

Hot Artichoke Dip

If you're having friends over at the last minute or just need to keep your hungry belly at bay until dinner is ready, this is a dependably delicious snack. Most of the ingredients are pantry staples, too! If you plan on eating artichokes more often—and you just might after diving into this dip—stock up on the frozen version, as canned artichokes can be high in sodium.

SERVES 8

1 cup gluten-free light mayonnaise
1 cup grated Parmesan cheese
1 cup canned or frozen artichoke hearts, drained, well rinsed, and chopped
2 garlic cloves, chopped
½ teaspoon gluten-free paprika
¼ teaspoon freshly ground black pepper
1 5-ounce box gluten-free crackers

Looking to get more fiber in your diet? Artichokes are a fiber all-star.

1. Preheat the oven to 425°F.

2. Place the mayonnaise, Parmesan, artichokes, garlic, paprika, and black pepper in a large bowl. Stir well to combine.

3. Transfer the artichoke mixture to an 8 × 8-inch baking dish, and bake for 20 to 25 minutes, until it is hot and bubbly. Serve immediately, with crackers.

Nachos and Guacamole

*Cool and creamy sour cream with nachos is a must for me. But beware:
As with "light" butter, some light sour cream is thickened with
modified food starch (i.e., gluten-based stabilizers) because it contains
less fat. Be sure to double-check your source.*

SERVES 8

Guacamole

4 large ripe avocados, preferably Hass
½ teaspoon sea salt, plus more if needed
3 ripe tomatoes, seeded and finely chopped
¼ cup minced red onion
2 jalapeños, seeded and finely chopped
3 tablespoons minced fresh cilantro

Nachos

I tablespoon olive oil
I pound ground beef
I tablespoon gluten-free mild chili powder
I tablespoon gluten-free ground cumin
I tablespoon cornstarch
½ teaspoon salt
2 large tomatoes, diced (about 2 cups)
Nonstick cooking spray
I 13-ounce bag gluten-free tortilla chips
½ cup pickled jalapeño slices
I cup shredded sharp cheddar cheese
I cup shredded Monterey Jack or pepper Jack cheese

Elisabeth Hasselbeck

1 cup gluten-free prepared salsa, for serving

1 cup gluten-free light sour cream, for serving

1. Prepare the guacamole: Cut the avocados in half, remove the pits, and scoop the flesh into a large wooden or metal bowl. Add the sea salt and mash with the back of a wooden spoon until the desired texture is reached—I like mine a bit chunky. Stir in the finely chopped tomatoes, onion, jalapeños, and cilantro. Taste, and add more salt if needed. To keep the guacamole for up to 3 hours, cover the surface of the dip directly with plastic wrap and store it in the refrigerator.

2. Make the nacho filling: Heat a large skillet over high heat and add the oil. Add the ground beef and cook, stirring occasionally, until it is browned, 3 to 4 minutes. Sprinkle the chili, cumin, and cornstarch over the beef. Add the salt, diced tomatoes, and ¼ cup of water. Cook for 2 to 3 minutes more, until the tomatoes start to break apart and a thick sauce forms.

3. Preheat the oven to 400°F.

4. Coat a rimmed baking sheet or a large ovenproof platter with a thin layer of cooking spray. Spread the tortilla chips out on the baking sheet. Spoon the filling over the tortilla chips, and sprinkle with the jalapeños and cheeses. Bake for 5 to 8 minutes, or until the cheeses have melted. Serve immediately with the guacamole, salsa, and sour cream.

Need to feed a crowd?

Whether for a baby shower brunch, a holiday buffet, or a game day grazing table, I have found that in addition to any of the appetizers in this chapter, the following recipes from other categories in this book—doubled or tripled, depending on how many mouths you want to feed—are real crowd-pleasers, too.

Blueberry Waffles

Fruit Salad with Dreamy Whipped
    Topping

French Toast with Caramel Rum
    Bananas

Blueberry Muffins

Coconut Raspberry Muffins

Egg Muffins

Egg "Doll" Biscuits

Quinoa Salad

Rob the Cobb Skinny Salad

Yellow Birthday Cake or Classic
    Yellow Cupcakes

Banana Cream Pie

Blueberry-Raspberry Cobbler

Chocolate Almond Bark

Double Chocolate Brownies

Banana Bread

Chocolate Chip Cookies

Mini "Hello Mellow" Dogs

Creamy Cheesecake with Berry
    Topping

Tiramisu

Angel Food Cake with Mini
    Chocolate Chips

Orange Cream Cupcakes

Buckeyes

{ *Chapter 4* }

Mouthwatering
Main Meals

These family-friendly meals were born out of my determination to make food that my husband, Tim, and our kids will love and that I can actually eat. Whether your own or a loved one's gluten sensitivity has brought you to this book, my dearest hope is that you too will rekindle your love for eating great food and come back to many dishes you thought were off-limits. Uninteresting and uninspired gluten-free cooking is a thing of the past, and as you browse these flavorful recipes, you'll also find tips on how to change them up slightly to keep your meals interesting and fresh.

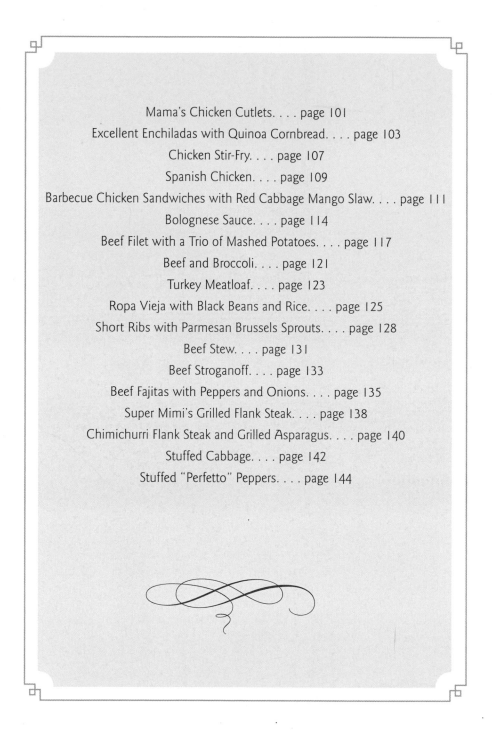

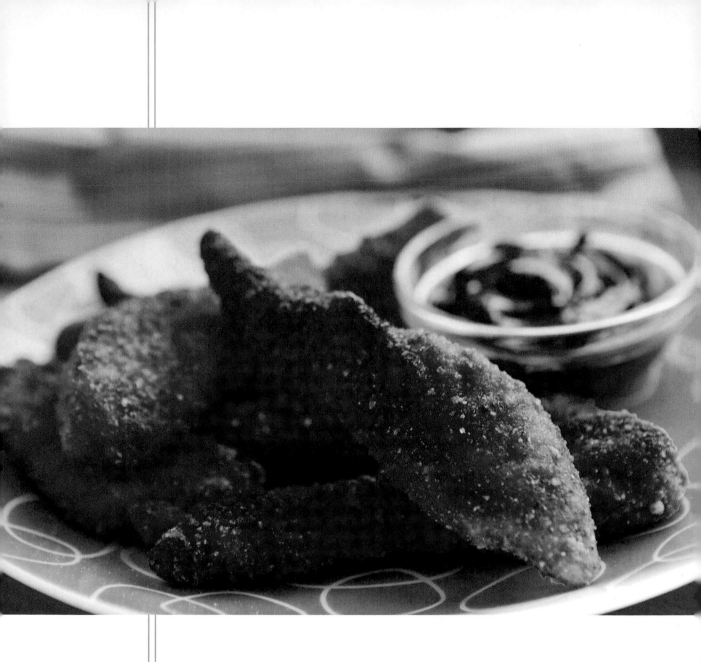

Elisabeth Hasselbeck

Kid-Pleasing Chicken Fingers

Paprika gives an appetizing golden hue to this kids' and take-out classic. Kids who have to eat g-free will be thrilled that these taste like the chicken fingers their friends can eat—and it's a bonus that they can help make them at home!

SERVES 4

½ teaspoon salt

1 pound chicken tenders

½ cup gluten-free rice crumbs

½ cup gluten-free corn crumbs

2 tablespoons grated Parmesan cheese

½ teaspoon gluten-free paprika

¼ teaspoon freshly ground black pepper

2 eggs

2 tablespoons olive oil

For a perky flavor lift, add ½ teaspoon of Italian seasoning to the crumb mix. I call this variation "Herby" chicken fingers and sometimes serve them with a side of warm marinara sauce and a melted slice of mozzarella cheese. Top with some grated Parmesan cheese and you've turned them into a chicken Parmesan dinner!

1. Preheat the oven to 400°F.

2. Sprinkle ¼ teaspoon of the salt over the chicken tenders.

3. Place the rice crumbs, corn crumbs, Parmesan, paprika, black pepper, and remaining ¼ teaspoon salt in a shallow bowl; mix with your fingertips until well combined. Place the eggs in a shallow bowl and whisk thoroughly. Dip the chicken tenders, one at a time, into the eggs to coat them, and then press them into the crumb mixture.

4. Heat a large ovenproof skillet over high heat, and add the olive oil. When the oil is hot, carefully add the chicken fingers.

Reduce the heat to medium and cook, turning them over once, until both sides are golden, about 4 minutes. Then slide the skillet into the oven and bake for 5 minutes, or until the chicken is cooked through. Let the chicken fingers cool for 2 minutes before serving.

Elisabeth Hasselbeck

Jalapeño and Hot Chile Chicken Fingers

Many jalapeño seasonings on the market already contain a good amount of salt, but if your g-free brand happens to be salt-free, add ½ teaspoon salt to your crumb mixture. Chipotle seasoning works equally well, and if you want to go atomic hot, use chipotle plus an extra teaspoon of crushed red pepper flakes.

SERVES 4

¼ teaspoon salt
I pound chicken tenders
½ cup gluten-free rice crumbs
½ cup gluten-free corn crumbs
I teaspoon jalapeño seasoning salt
½ teaspoon crushed gluten-free red pepper flakes
¼ teaspoon freshly ground black pepper
2 eggs
2 tablespoons olive oil

1. Preheat the oven to 400°F.

2. Sprinkle the salt over the chicken tenders.

3. Place the rice crumbs, corn crumbs, jalapeño seasoning, red pepper flakes, and black pepper in a shallow bowl; mix with your fingertips until well combined. Place the eggs in a shallow bowl and whisk thoroughly. Dip the chicken tenders, one at a time, into the eggs to coat them, and then press them into the crumb mixture.

4. Heat a large ovenproof skillet over high heat, and add the olive oil. When the oil is hot, carefully add the chicken fingers. Reduce the heat to medium and cook, turning them over once, until both sides are golden, about 4 minutes. Then slide the skillet into the oven and bake for 5 minutes, or until the chicken is cooked through. Let the chicken fingers cool for 2 minutes before serving.

Basic Roast Chicken

Start the week off right with this warm Sunday-night dinner. Make two and you are off to an even better start with fantastic leftovers for the rest of the week, either as a perfect meal once more or repurposed into great sandwiches and salads!

SERVES 4

1 3-pound chicken
½ teaspoon salt
¼ teaspoon freshly ground black pepper
2 teaspoons canola oil

1. Preheat the oven to 350°F.

2. Sprinkle the chicken with the salt and black pepper. Heat a medium ovenproof skillet over high heat and add the canola oil. Carefully place the chicken, breast side down, in the skillet and reduce the heat to medium. Brown for 3 to 4 minutes without turning.

3. Turn the chicken over and brown for 1 minute more. Then slide the skillet into the oven and roast until the chicken is no longer pink at the leg joints and the juices run clear, about 1½ hours. (An instant-read thermometer inserted near the leg joint, but not touching bone, should read 170°F.)

4. Transfer the chicken to a cutting board and let it rest for at least 15 minutes to allow the juices to redistribute. Then carve the chicken and serve immediately.

Not enough leftover chicken to make a complete meal? Don't toss it; stir it into my Classic Chicken Noodle Soup (page 91).

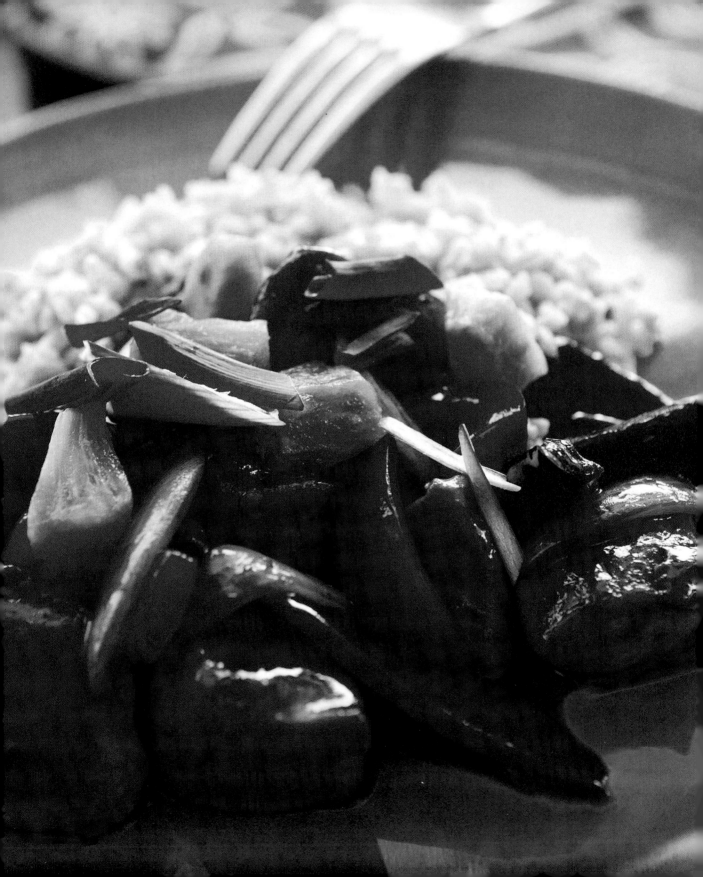

Sweet and Sour Chicken

This deliciously g-free version is so good, you may never order out

again. Add fried rice and chopsticks, and you are good to go!

SERVES 4

¼ cup gluten-free chicken broth (see page 92 for my homemade version)

3 tablespoons gluten-free soy sauce

2 tablespoons gluten-free ketchup

I tablespoon gluten-free rice vinegar

I tablespoon cornstarch

I tablespoon gluten-free light brown sugar

2 tablespoons canola oil

2 pounds boneless, skinless chicken breasts, cut into I½-inch chunks

2 bell peppers (green, red, yellow, or a combination),
    cut into I-inch pieces

½ sweet white onion, such as Vidalia or Walla Walla, diced

2 large carrots, thinly sliced

2 garlic cloves, thinly sliced

I cup diced fresh pineapple; or I cup canned diced pineapple in
    natural juice, drained

8 scallions, cut into I-inch pieces, using both white and green parts

2 cups cooked gluten-free short-grain brown rice, for serving

Compared to your average restaurant version, this recipe saves you about 10 grams of fat, and it's naturally MSG-free.

1. Place the chicken broth, soy sauce, ketchup, rice vinegar, cornstarch, and brown sugar in a small bowl. Whisk until well combined. Set aside.

2. Heat a large skillet over high heat. Add 1 tablespoon of the canola oil and the chicken. Cook the chicken, turning the pieces once or twice, until they are browned on the outside, 2 to 3 minutes. Transfer the chicken to a plate.

3. Add the remaining 1 tablespoon canola oil to the skillet along with the bell peppers, onion, carrots, and garlic. Cook, stirring often, until the peppers and onions start to soften, 2 to 3 minutes.

4. Return the chicken and any accumulated juices to the skillet, and reduce the heat to low. Stir the chicken broth mixture and add it to the skillet. Cook, stirring often, for 2 minutes or until a thick sauce forms and the chicken is cooked through. Top with the pineapple or stir the pineapple in. Sprinkle with the scallions and serve immediately with the rice.

Elisabeth Hasselbeck

Classic Chicken Noodle Soup

Chicken soup is like a big food hug. My mom has never failed to have this soup on hand for me whenever I needed comforting—the warm, delicious bowl always brings a smile to my face. Nutritionally, the escarole adds folate and vitamin A, and I like to serve the soup to my family during the winter months so we can all better handle the cold weather or our sniffles.

SERVES 6

2 bone-in, skin-on chicken breasts (about 1¼ pounds)

½ teaspoon salt

¼ teaspoon freshly ground black pepper

1 tablespoon olive oil

4 carrots, thinly sliced

2 celery stalks, finely chopped

2 leeks, white portion only, halved, chopped, and well rinsed

1 quart gluten-free chicken broth (see recipe page 92)

¼ cup minced fresh flat-leaf parsley

1 teaspoon fresh thyme leaves

1 bay leaf

1 pound escarole, chopped

½ pound brown rice, quinoa, or gluten-free noodles, cooked according to the package instructions

It's best to cook the rice, quinoa, or noodles separately and then add them just before serving—they can become mushy if cooked directly in the soup.

1. Sprinkle the chicken with the salt and black pepper. Heat a large stockpot over high heat. Add the olive oil and the chicken breasts, skin side down. Scatter the carrots, celery, and leeks around the chicken. Reduce the heat to medium and cook, stirring occasionally, until the chicken begins to brown lightly and the vegetables soften, 4 to 5 minutes.

2. Remove the chicken from the pot, and remove and discard the skin and bones. Return the chicken meat to the pot and add the chicken broth, parsley, thyme, and bay leaf. Bring to a steady simmer and cook for 10 minutes.

3. Remove the stockpot from the heat, and let the chicken finish poaching in the liquid for 25 minutes. Take out the bay leaf, and add the escarole during the last 5 minutes.

4. Stir in the brown rice, quinoa, or noodles. Serve immediately, or let cool and then store in an airtight container in the refrigerator for up to 3 days. Add the brown rice, quinoa, or noodles in before warming again.

Homemade Chicken Broth *Store-bought broths often list a number of confusing ingredients, and too often gluten can hide therein. Preparing your own broth does take a little effort, but the results are beyond what you could ever buy—and you can be sure it's gluten-free!*

MAKES 2 QUARTS

2 pounds chicken legs (thighs and drumsticks, skin on)
½ teaspoon salt
¼ teaspoon freshly ground black pepper
1 tablespoon olive oil
1 large yellow onion, chopped
2 carrots, quartered
2 celery stalks, quartered
4 sprigs of flat-leaf parsley (stems and leaves)

Elisabeth Hasselbeck

2 bay leaves

2 teaspoons whole black peppercorns

1. Sprinkle the chicken legs with the salt and black pepper. Heat a large stockpot over medium-high heat, and add the olive oil. Add the chicken legs, skin side down. Scatter the onion, carrots, and celery around the chicken. Cook, turning occasionally, until the chicken begins to brown, 8 to 10 minutes.

2. Tuck the parsley and bay leaves around the chicken, and cover the chicken with 2½ quarts (10 cups) of water. Add the peppercorns. Bring to a steady simmer and cook for 1 hour, occasionally skimming the top of the broth to remove any white foam that forms.

3. Remove the chicken legs from the pot, reserving the meat for another recipe. Strain the broth into storage containers and discard the vegetables. Let the broth cool to room temperature. Then cover and refrigerate for up to 1 week or freeze for up to 3 months.

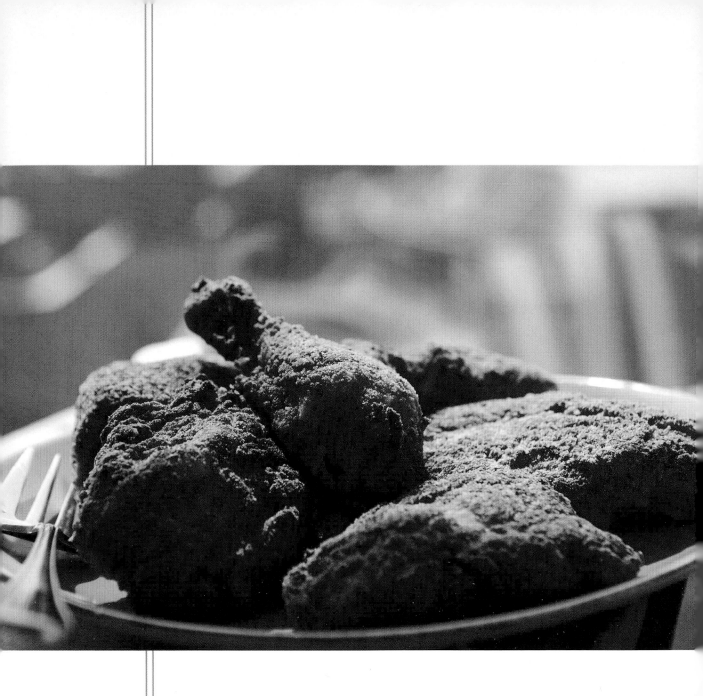

Elisabeth Hasselbeck

Buttermilk Chicken

This gluten-free gourmet chicken will literally melt in your mouth! It's a great choice to serve hot for a special occasion, but it also tastes great at room temperature and even cold, making it the ideal main course for a picnic or family get-together.

SERVES 4

4 skinless, boneless chicken breast halves (about 2 pounds total)
2 garlic cloves, minced
1 tablespoon finely chopped fresh rosemary
1½ cups low-fat buttermilk
1 egg
½ cup brown rice flour
¾ cup crushed gluten-free cornflakes
2 tablespoons finely grated Parmesan cheese
2 teaspoons gluten-free paprika
1 teaspoon gluten-free garlic powder
1 teaspoon salt
¼ teaspoon freshly ground black pepper
¼ cup canola oil
2 tablespoons chopped fresh flat-leaf parsley

1. Place the chicken breasts, garlic, and rosemary in a bowl, and add 1 cup of the buttermilk. Cover and refrigerate for at least 1 hour or up to 8 hours.

2. In a shallow bowl, beat the egg with a fork until blended. Then add the remaining ½ cup buttermilk and the brown rice flour, and beat until a thick batter forms. On a plate, mix together the cornflakes, Parmesan, paprika, garlic powder, salt, and black pepper.

3. Using tongs, lift each chicken breast from the buttermilk and dip into the egg mixture. Then dip each piece one at a time into the cornflake mixture. When all the chicken pieces are coated, refrigerate them for 30 minutes to help the cornflake coating adhere.

4. Preheat the oven to 400°F.

5. Place a deep skillet over high heat, and add the canola oil. When the oil is hot (a tiny piece of chicken dipped into the hot oil will sizzle as soon as it's added), add half the chicken pieces without crowding the pan. Working in batches, fry the chicken, turning the pieces as needed, until they are well browned on all sides, about 10 minutes total. As soon as the chicken breasts are browned, transfer them to a baking sheet.

6. Transfer the baking sheet to the oven, and bake until the chicken is opaque throughout and the juices run clear, 25 to 30 minutes.

7. Arrange the chicken on a serving platter, garnish with the parsley, and serve warm or at room temperature.

Elisabeth Hasselbeck

Tequila Lime Chicken Salad

This is one fresh salad that will become a seasonal staple—the perfect recipe for a lazy summer dinner or for lunch with friends.

SERVES 4

½ cup gold tequila
I cup freshly squeezed lime juice (from 5 to 6 limes)
½ cup freshly squeezed orange juice (from 2 oranges)
I tablespoon gluten-free chili powder
I tablespoon minced fresh jalapeño (from I pepper, seeded)
3 garlic cloves, minced
Salt and freshly ground black pepper
4 skinless, boneless chicken breasts
canola oil, for the grill

Dressing
½ cup orange juice
¼ cup chopped chili en adobo
3 tablespoons olive oil

2 cups mesclun greens
2 cups finely shredded red cabbage

1. Combine the tequila, lime juice, orange juice, chili powder, jalapeño, garlic, 1 teaspoon salt, and 1 teaspoon black pepper in a large bowl, and stir well. Add the chicken breasts, cover, and refrigerate overnight.

2. Heat a grill with coals and brush the rack with canola oil to prevent the chicken from sticking.

3. Remove the chicken breasts from the marinade, season them well with salt and black pepper, and grill them for about 5 minutes, until nicely browned.

4. Turn the chicken over and cook for another 10 minutes, until just cooked through. Transfer the chicken to a plate and let it rest for 5 minutes before slicing.

5. Prepare the dressing: Place the orange juice, chili en adobo, and olive oil in a blender. Blend until smooth. Set aside.

6. Place the mesclun greens and cabbage in a large bowl or on a platter. Slice the chicken and arrange it over the greens. Drizzle with the dressing and serve immediately.

Chicken Marsala

Another classic Italian meal, made g-free! Easy to put together, this super-rich chicken and flavorful sauce won't disappoint. Leftovers make a satisfying toasted sandwich (try topping it with a slice of Swiss cheese).

SERVE 4

1 teaspoon salt
4 chicken cutlets (thinly sliced chicken breast; about ¾ pound total)
½ cup brown rice flour
¼ cup tapioca starch
2 tablespoons olive oil
10 ounces Cremini or white button mushrooms
1 small sweet onion or 2 shallots, finely chopped
½ cup sweet Marsala wine
½ cup gluten-free chicken broth
2 tablespoons heavy cream
2 tablespoons chopped fresh flat-leaf parsley

1. Sprinkle the salt over the chicken. Place the brown rice flour and tapioca starch on a sheet of wax paper and mix them together with your fingers. Dredge the chicken cutlets in the flour mixture and set aside.

2. Heat a large deep skillet over high heat. Add 1 tablespoon of the olive oil, the mushrooms, and the onions or shallots. Cook for 2 to 3 minutes, until the mushrooms start to soften. Transfer the mushroom mixture to a plate.

3. Add the remaining 1 tablespoon olive oil and the chicken to the skillet. Cook, turning the cutlets once, until they are browned on both sides, 2 to 3 minutes. Add the Marsala and cook for 2 to 3 minutes, until the liquid has reduced by half. Add the chicken broth and cook for 3 minutes more, until the liquid has reduced by half. Return the mushroom mixture to the skillet and remove from the heat. Pour in the cream and stir to combine. Sprinkle with the parsley and serve immediately.

Mama's Chicken Cutlets

I can still remember chicken cutlets, hot from the pan, lined up on paper towels at my grandmother's house, and now I can make them g-free! They make a great dinner when you add a veggie side dish like Parmesan Brussels Sprouts (page 128), and are equally as good when served in a sandwich the next day. I'm all for cooking once and enjoying twice, so double up on the numbers below, and you will be glad the next day when a cutlet makes its way into your paper bag lunch.

SERVES 4

Four slices of g-free bread will yield about 2 cups of crumbs.

4 skinless, boneless chicken cutlets (about ¾ pound total)
½ teaspoon salt
¼ teaspoon freshly ground black pepper
½ cup brown rice flour
2 eggs
I cup gluten-free bread crumbs
¼ cup grated Parmesan cheese
I teaspoon grated lemon zest
I teaspoon dried oregano
I teaspoon gluten-free paprika
2 tablespoons olive oil

1. Line a baking sheet with wax paper or aluminum foil.
2. Using a flat meat pounder, pound each chicken cutlet until it is flattened to an even thickness of about ½ inch. Sprinkle the chicken with ¼ teaspoon of the salt and the black pepper.

3. Spread the brown rice flour out on a sheet of wax paper. In a shallow bowl, whisk the eggs. In a second shallow bowl, stir the bread crumbs, Parmesan, lemon zest, oregano, and paprika together with a fork. Dip each chicken cutlet into the flour, coating it evenly and shaking off the excess flour. Then dip the chicken into the eggs, coating it evenly and allowing the excess to drip off. Finally, coat it evenly with the bread-crumb mixture. Transfer the chicken cutlets to the prepared baking sheet.

4. Line another baking sheet or a large plate with paper towels.

5. In a large skillet over medium heat, warm the olive oil until it is very hot but not smoking, about 10 seconds. Add the chicken and cook, adjusting the heat as needed, until golden brown, about 4 minutes. Turn the chicken over and cook until browned on the other side, 3 to 4 minutes more. Transfer the chicken to the paper towels and sprinkle with the remaining ¼ teaspoon salt. Serve immediately.

Elisabeth Hasselbeck

Excellent Enchiladas with Quinoa Cornbread

My husband, Tim, gave this recipe its name—which tells you something about the deliciousness factor! I think the salsa verde makes the enchiladas taste unique and refreshing. They can also be made with red enchilada sauce, but be sure to check the label because some red enchilada sauces do contain gluten.

SERVES 8

Nonstick cooking spray

1 tablespoon canola oil

2 skinless, boneless chicken breasts, cut into strips

½ red onion, chopped

2 garlic cloves, thinly sliced

1 teaspoon salt

1 small head broccoli, florets chopped, stems discarded

2 16-ounce jars gluten-free salsa verde or 4 cups homemade Salsa Verde (see page 147)

12 5-inch gluten-free corn tortillas

2 cups shredded Monterey Jack, pepper Jack, or white cheddar cheese

1. Preheat the oven to 400°F.

2. Coat a 9 × 13-inch casserole with nonstick spray.

3. Heat a large skillet over high heat and add the canola oil. Add the chicken strips, onion, and garlic, and reduce the heat to medium. Sprinkle with the salt. Cook, stirring often, until the onion softens and the chicken starts to brown, 4 to 5 minutes.

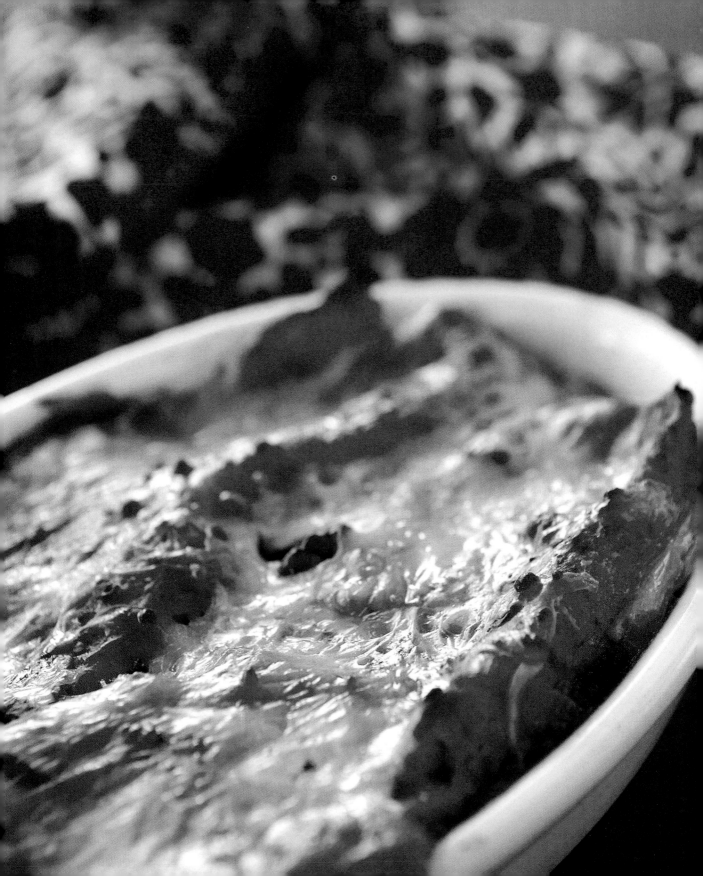

Add the broccoli and 1 cup of the salsa verde. Cook, stirring often, for 1 minute more, or until the broccoli starts to soften. Set aside.

4. Pour the remaining 1 cup of salsa verde from the first jar into the prepared casserole, and spread it out evenly. Pour the other jar of salsa verde (2 cups) into a shallow bowl. Dip a tortilla into the bowl of salsa verde to moisten both sides, and then layer ¼ cup of the filling and 2 tablespoons of the cheese in the center of the tortilla. Pull the edges of the tortilla together so that they overlap a bit, and place it, seam side down, in the casserole. Repeat with the remaining tortillas. Spoon what's left of the salsa verde in the shallow bowl over the enchiladas, and sprinkle the remaining cheese down the center of the casserole dish.

5. Cover the casserole with aluminum foil and bake for 30 minutes.

6. Remove the foil and continue baking until the cheese is bubbling and lightly browned, about 20 minutes. Remove the casserole from the oven and let it stand for 10 minutes before serving.

Quinoa Cornbread

Quinoa gives this cheesy, spicy, Southwestern side dish its moistness—no one will believe it's g-free. It's so good, in fact, that I like to sneak the first piece just to ensure that I get my share!

SERVES 12

Nonstick cooking spray
1 cup brown rice flour
¾ cup gluten-free fine cornmeal
1 tablespoon baking powder

½ teaspoon xanthan gum

½ teaspoon salt

1 cup cooked quinoa

¾ cup 2% milk

1 egg

2 scallions, thinly sliced, using both white and green parts

2 jalapeños, seeded and chopped

¼ cup honey

½ cup grated pepper Jack cheese

½ cup fresh or frozen corn kernels (defrosted if frozen)

1. Preheat the oven to 400°F. Coat an 8 × 8-inch baking pan with cooking spray.

2. Place the brown rice flour, cornmeal, baking powder, xanthan gum, salt, and quinoa in a large bowl, and combine well. Add the milk, egg, scallions, jalapeños, honey, and corn kernels and mix just until combined—there might be some dry spots. Transfer the mixture to the prepared baking pan and sprinkle the cheese over the top.

3. Bake for 12 to 14 minutes, until the edges are beginning to brown lightly and the cheese has melted. Let the cornbread cool in the pan for 2 minutes before cutting into squares; then enjoy. (Let any extra cool completely before storing it in an airtight container at room temperature for up to 3 days.)

Chicken Stir-Fry

I find that a stir-fry works well toward the end of the week when my produce is running low and I have what I call "lonely veggies." Those stragglers find a nice home in this dish.

SERVES 4

2 skinless boneless chicken breast fillets, cut into thin strips

¼ cup gluten-free soy sauce

2 garlic cloves, minced

½ cup gluten-free chicken broth or water

2 teaspoons cornstarch

2 tablespoons grated peeled fresh ginger

1 tablespoon Asian sesame oil

2 teaspoons granulated sugar

2 tablespoons canola oil, or as needed

¼ head red or green cabbage, thinly sliced

2 carrots, thinly sliced

2 jalapeños, seeded and finely diced, or 1 green bell pepper, seeded and finely diced

10 ounces shiitake mushrooms, thinly sliced

1 cup gluten-free short-grain brown rice, cooked according to the package instructions, for serving

Stir-fries are a great way to get your protein needs and vital veggies in a one-pan preparation.

1. In a medium bowl, toss the chicken with the soy sauce and garlic. Set aside.

2. Place the chicken broth or water, cornstarch, ginger, sesame oil, and sugar in a small bowl and whisk to combine. Set aside.

3. Place a large wok or skillet over high heat, and add 1 tablespoon of the canola oil. Add the chicken and marinade, and stir-fry for 1 minute. Transfer it to a plate. Add the remaining 1 tablespoon canola oil to the skillet, and add the cabbage, carrots, jalapeños or bell peppers, and mushrooms. Cook for 2 to 3 minutes, stirring often.

4. Reduce the heat to low. Whisk the sauce mixture and pour it into the wok. Add the reserved chicken. Cook for 2 to 3 minutes, or just until the liquid comes to a boil and the chicken is cooked through.

5. Spoon the rice onto individual plates, and top with the stir-fry and sauce.

Elisabeth Hasselbeck

Spanish Chicken

I can easily get in a chicken dinner rut, making the same handful of meals over and over again. If you want to shake things up for your next dinner, give this a try. Your taste buds will be alive and happy with the first bite!

SERVES 4

1 tablespoon olive oil

4 bone-in, skin-on chicken breast halves

1 teaspoon salt

¼ teaspoon freshly ground black pepper

1 medium yellow onion, chopped

2 garlic cloves, finely chopped

1 bay leaf

½ cup cured, pitted black olives

4 ripe tomatoes (about 1 pound total), coarsely chopped

½ red onion, minced

Juice of 2 limes

1 jalapeño, seeded and diced

1 teaspoon chopped fresh oregano

¼ teaspoon granulated sugar

1 13-ounce bag gluten-free tortilla chips

Cooking chicken on the bone helps to keep the meat insulated and moist.

1. Heat a large stockpot over medium-high heat and add the olive oil. Sprinkle the chicken with ½ teaspoon of the salt and black pepper, and place it, skin side down, in the stockpot. Add the yellow onion, garlic, and bay leaf. Cook for 2 to 3 minutes, until the onion starts to soften and the chicken starts to brown. Add the olives and enough water to cover the chicken.

2. Bring to a boil, and then immediately reduce to a simmer and cover the pot. Cook for 20 to 25 minutes, until the chicken is cooked through to the bone and no longer pink.

3. Meanwhile, prepare the salsa: Place the tomatoes, red onion, lime juice, jalapeño, oregano, sugar, and remaining ½ teaspoon salt in a bowl, and toss to combine.

4. Once the chicken is cooked, remove it from the pot and re-serve the olives. When the chicken is cool enough to handle, re-move and discard the skin and bones. Shred the meat and place it on a platter. Layer the olives on top of the chicken. Spoon the salsa over the chicken, and serve immediately with tortilla chips.

Barbecue Chicken Sandwiches with Red Cabbage Mango Slaw

This is the perfect picnic sandwich. You can use tortillas as the "bread" or try serving the chicken on mini buns (like sliders) with the slaw on the side. The first time I made this recipe for Tim, he didn't speak to me . . . until he was finished!

SERVES 4

Red Cabbage Mango Slaw
¼ cup gluten-free light mayonnaise

2 tablespoons plain 2% Greek yogurt

1 tablespoon honey

1 tablespoon red wine vinegar

¼ teaspoon salt

⅛ teaspoon freshly ground black pepper

½ head red cabbage, shredded

2 medium mangoes, peeled, pitted, and shredded

Barbecue Chicken
1 tablespoon olive or canola oil

1 large onion, chopped

2 bone-in, skin-on chicken breasts

1 cup prepared gluten-free barbecue sauce

2 tablespoons honey

2 tablespoons salted butter

8 5-inch gluten-free corn tortillas, warmed, or 4 gluten-free sandwich buns, for serving

You can prepare this dish up to 2 days in advance. Just store the chicken and the slaw in separate airtight containers, and refrigerate until ready to use.

1. Make the slaw: Place the mayonnaise, yogurt, honey, vinegar, salt, and black pepper in a large bowl and whisk until well combined. Add the red cabbage and the mangoes. Toss to coat. Cover and refrigerate until ready to serve.

2. Prepare the chicken: Heat a medium saucepan over high heat. Add the olive or canola oil, onion, and the chicken breasts, skin side down. Reduce the heat to medium and cook for 3 to 4 minutes, as the chicken browns. Add the barbecue sauce and the honey. Cover, and reduce to a simmer. Cook for 35 to 40 minutes, until the chicken is cooked through.

3. Remove the chicken from the sauce, and remove and discard the skin and bones. Shred the meat with a fork, and return it along with the butter to the sauce, and stir well to coat.

4. Serve with the slaw on tortillas or mini buns.

Elisabeth Hasselbeck

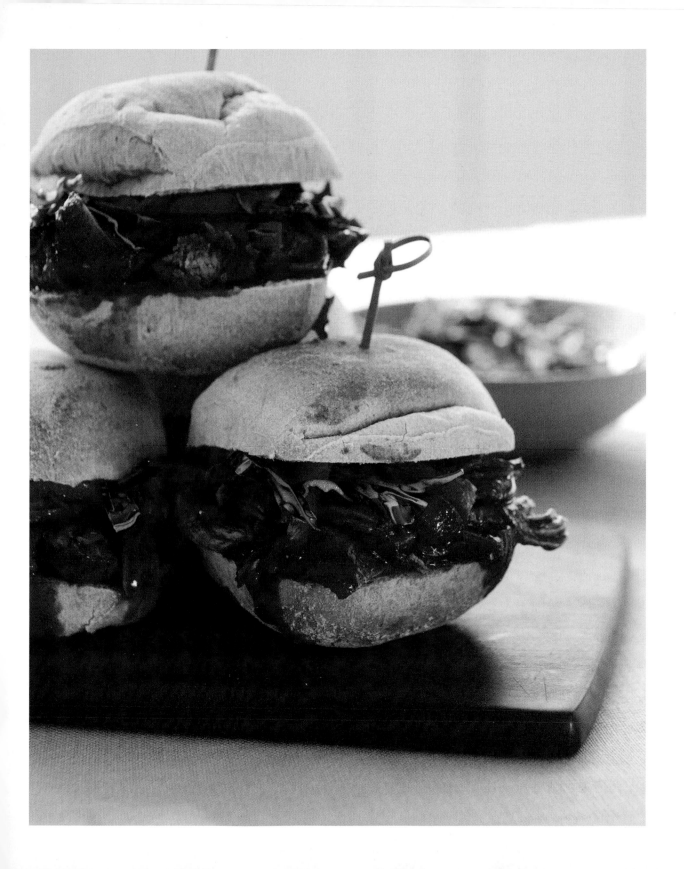

Bolognese Sauce

Want to show off your deliciously gluten-free skills? This dish will have them absolutely fooled! Pancetta gives the meat sauce the rich smoky taste that meat-lovers clamor for. For holidays or large dinner parties, the sauce can be made several days ahead of time and refrigerated.

SERVES 12

2 tablespoons olive oil
1 pound ground pork
1 pound ground veal
1 teaspoon salt
¼ teaspoon freshly ground black pepper
1 large yellow or red onion, finely chopped
3 carrots, finely chopped
2 celery stalks, finely chopped
1 2-ounce slice pancetta, chopped (about ½ cup)
3 tablespoons gluten-free tomato paste
1 cup dry white wine
4 cups gluten-free beef broth, at room temperature
1 pound gluten-free short-cut pasta, such as penne or rigatoni
¼ cup half-and-half
1 cup shredded Parmesan cheese

1. Heat 1 tablespoon of the olive oil in a large stockpot over medium-high heat. Sprinkle the pork and veal with the salt and black pepper. Add both meats to the stockpot and cook without stirring for about 1 minute, until the edges start to brown. Stir

Elisabeth Hasselbeck

the meat once or twice, and continue to brown it for 2 to 3 minutes more. Transfer the meat to a plate.

2. Place the same stockpot over medium heat, and add the remaining 1 tablespoon olive oil along with the onion, carrots, celery, and pancetta. Cook for 4 to 5 minutes, until the vegetables start to soften. Add the tomato paste and cook for 1 minute more, stirring often so the tomato paste coats the vegetables.

3. Return the meat to the stockpot. Add the wine, and cook for 5 minutes, until the liquid has reduced by half. Add 2 cups of the beef broth, stir well, and bring to a gentle boil. Then cover the pot, reduce the heat to a slow simmer, and cook for 2½ to 3 hours, checking the pot every 30 minutes and adding more broth as needed to keep the meat covered with liquid as it cooks. After most of the broth has been absorbed and a thick rich sauce has formed, remove the pot from the heat.

4. Bring a large pot of salted water to a boil, add the pasta, and cook according to the package instructions.

5. Reserving 1 cup of the cooking water, drain the pasta. Transfer the drained pasta and the reserved cooking water to the stockpot and heat over low heat for 1 minute, tossing the pasta with the sauce. Remove the stockpot from the heat, add the half-and-half, and stir well. Serve immediately, with the Parmesan alongside.

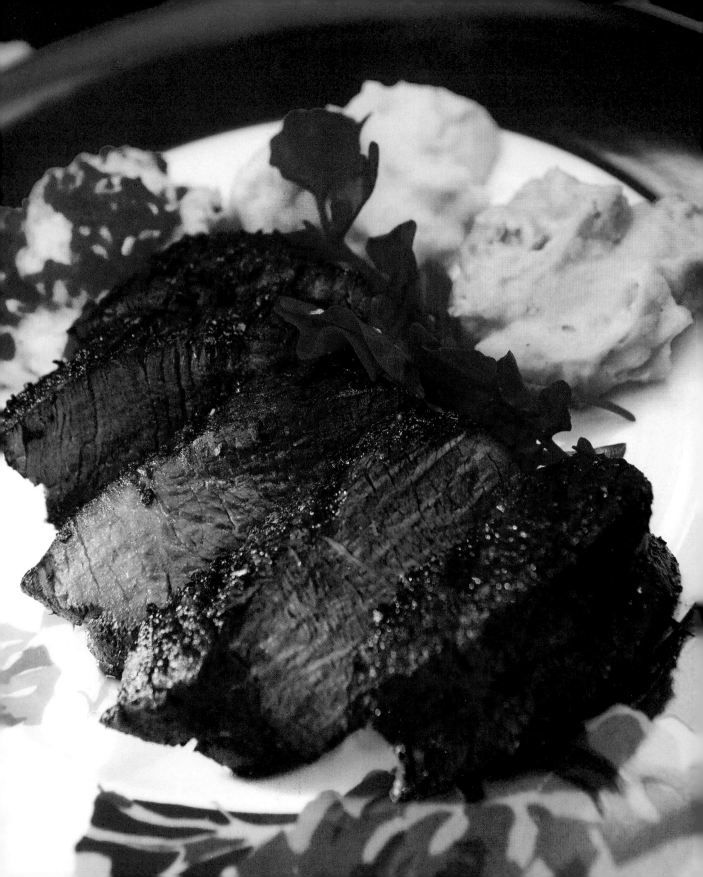

Beef Filet with a Trio of Mashed Potatoes

The magic of this recipe comes from searing and then roasting the meat. If only I had known about that simple two-step process earlier, I would not have charred so many great cuts of meat in the broiler! Now I not only enjoy the sit-down, I confidently love the process of getting there.

SERVES 4

4 filets mignons, each about ¼ pound and 1½ inches thick
4 teaspoons gluten-free steak rub, such as Montreal Steak Seasoning
1 tablespoon canola oil

Top your steaks with caramelized onions from my pork chop recipe (see page 156) or with creamy chipotle mayo (page 37).

1. Season each filet on both sides with 1 teaspoon of the steak rub. Let stand at room temperature for 30 minutes.

2. Preheat the oven to 450°F.

3. Place an ovenproof grill pan over medium-high heat, and warm the canola oil on it until it is almost smoking. Place the filets in the pan and cook, turning once, until browned, about 2 minutes per side. Then transfer the pan to the oven and roast until an instant-read thermometer inserted into the center of the filets registers 130°F for medium-rare (or from 7 minutes for rare to 12 minutes for medium).

4. Transfer the filets to a platter, cover loosely with aluminum foil, and let rest for 5 minutes to allow the juices to redistribute before serving.

Trio of Mashed Potatoes

Comfort, comfort, comfort! Three versions of scrumptious mashed potatoes to please everyone's taste buds: the classic-ista, the heat-seeker, and the cheese-lover, can all sit down to their favorite meal together. I have been known to sneak into the fridge for spoonfuls when nighttime snack cravings hit. I always hope there's enough left over!

Classic-ista

SERVES 4

As potatoes cool, their starch congeals. Always mash potatoes when they are piping hot to get the best texture and taste.

1 pound boiling potatoes, such as Red Bliss or Yukon Gold, cubed
½ cup gluten-free light sour cream
4 tablespoons (½ stick) salted butter at room temperature
½ teaspoon salt

1. Place the potatoes in a medium saucepan filled with cold water. Bring to a boil over high heat. Reduce the heat to a simmer and cook for 20 to 25 minutes, until the potatoes are fork-tender.

2. Drain the potatoes and place them in a large bowl. Add the sour cream, butter, and salt. Mash with a handheld potato masher. Serve immediately.

Elisabeth Hasselbeck

Wasabi Heat

SERVES 4

1 pound boiling potatoes, such as Red Bliss or Yukon Gold, cubed
½ cup gluten-free light sour cream
4 tablespoons (½ stick) salted butter
½ teaspoon salt
2 tablespoons gluten-free wasabi paste

1. Place the potatoes in a medium saucepan filled with cold water. Bring to a boil over high heat. Reduce the heat to a simmer and cook for 20 to 25 minutes, until the potatoes are fork-tender.

2. Drain the potatoes and place them in a large bowl. Add the sour cream, butter, salt, and wasabi. Mash with a handheld potato masher. Serve immediately.

Cheddar Love

SERVES 4

1 pound boiling potatoes, such as Red Bliss or Yukon Gold, cubed
1 cup finely grated cheddar cheese
½ cup gluten-free light sour cream
¼ cup grated Parmesan cheese
4 tablespoons (½ stick) salted butter at room temperature
½ teaspoon salt

1. Place the potatoes in a medium saucepan filled with cold water. Bring to a boil over high heat. Reduce the heat to a simmer and cook for 20 to 25 minutes, until the potatoes are fork-tender.

2. Drain the potatoes and place them in a large bowl. Add the cheddar, sour cream, Parmesan, butter, and salt. Mash with a handheld potato masher. Serve immediately.

Elisabeth Hasselbeck

Beef and Broccoli

This dish provides plenty of vitamin C and calcium from the broccoli, as well as fiber and a powerful punch of protein from the beans. Serve it over rice or g-free noodles for the ultimate feast.

SERVES 4

½ cup gluten-free beef broth
1 tablespoon gluten-free peanut butter
1 tablespoon gluten-free soy sauce
1 tablespoon gluten-free rice vinegar
2 teaspoons cornstarch
1 teaspoon granulated sugar
2 garlic cloves, minced
1 tablespoon canola oil
½ pound beef strips for stir-fry
1 head broccoli, cut into florets, thick stems discarded
1 tablespoon Asian sesame oil
1 15-ounce can black beans, drained and well rinsed

If you don't plan on eating this dish right away, steam the broccoli separately and let it cool before folding it in just before serving.

1. Place the beef broth, peanut butter, soy sauce, rice vinegar, cornstarch, sugar, and garlic in a bowl, and whisk until smooth. Set aside.

2. Heat the canola oil in a large skillet over high heat until it is hot but not smoking. Add the beef strips and cook, stirring often, until they just start to brown, 1 to 2 minutes. Using a slotted spoon, transfer the strips to a plate.

3. Add the broccoli and sesame oil to the skillet. Cook, stirring constantly, until golden, about 30 seconds. Reduce the heat to low and add ½ cup of water. Cover the skillet and cook until the mixture is dry and the broccoli is tender, about 2 minutes.

4. Stir the broth mixture, and add it to the skillet. Return the beef and any accumulated juices to the skillet along with the beans and cook, stirring often, until the beef is heated through, about 1 minute. Serve immediately.

Elisabeth Hasselbeck

Turkey Meatloaf

Turkey makes this delicious meatloaf a lot lower in fat than the usual beef and/or pork version. (There's no need to tell beef-lovers, because the soy sauce darkens the meat mixture!) Always a family favorite, it's a bona fide kid-taste-approved meal in my house . . . and it's fun for them to help with all of the ingredients and prep too!

SERVES 4

½ cup grated yellow squash
¼ cup gluten-free cornmeal
¼ cup 2% milk
3 tablespoons gluten-free soy sauce
1 pound ground dark turkey meat
1 egg
2 garlic cloves, minced
Nonstick cooking spray
½ cup gluten-free ketchup or barbecue sauce

1. Preheat the oven to 350°F.

2. Place the yellow squash, cornmeal, milk, and soy sauce in a large bowl, and stir well. Let the mixture rest for 15 minutes to allow the cornmeal to soak up some of the liquid. Then add the turkey, egg, and garlic. Mix well.

3. Spray a loaf pan with cooking spray and add the meat mixture to the pan, smoothing the surface. Top with the ketchup or barbecue sauce.

4. Bake for 45 to 50 minutes, until the meatloaf is no longer pink in the center (test by inserting a knife and looking). Let the meatloaf rest for 5 minutes before slicing and serving.

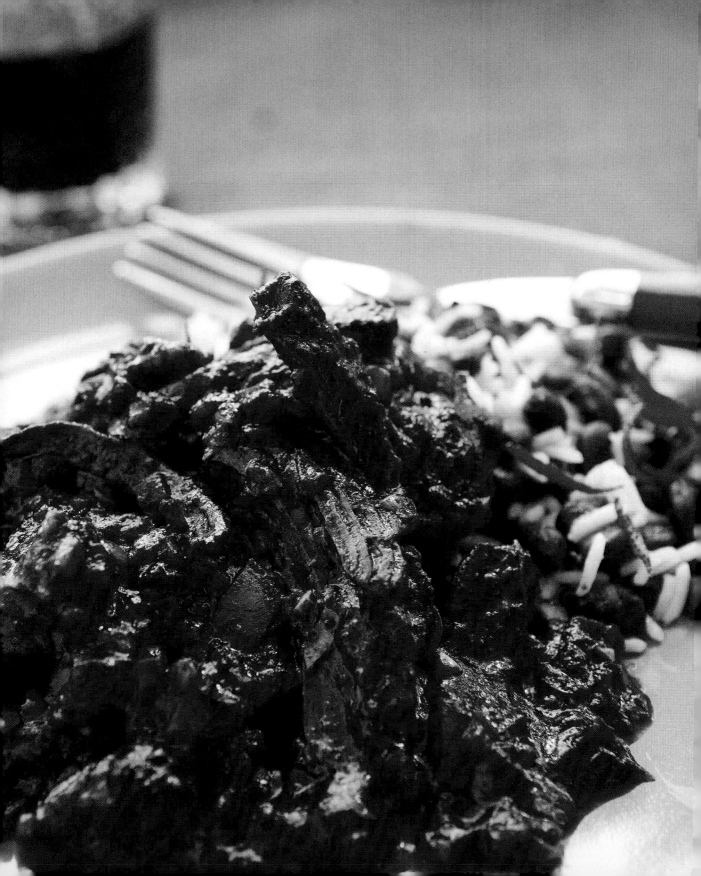

Ropa Vieja with Black Beans and Rice

 Ropa vieja *means "old clothes" in Spanish, which is fitting because the long, tender shreds of beef do* appetizingly *resemble twisted clothing. This dish reheats well, but be warned: there are rarely any leftovers in my experience! For variety, swap out the black beans and rice for mashed potatoes (see page 118).*

SERVES 8

Steak

1 large flank steak (2 pounds)
2 medium onions, coarsely chopped
2 carrots, coarsely chopped
3 celery stalks, coarsely chopped
2 bay leaves
1 teaspoon whole black peppercorns

Sauce

1 tablespoon olive oil
1 medium red onion, finely chopped
1 small green bell pepper, seeded and finely chopped
4 garlic cloves, minced
½ teaspoon salt
1 tablespoon gluten-free tomato paste
½ teaspoon gluten-free ground cumin
1 teaspoon dried oregano
1 28-ounce can chopped tomatoes with juices

Flank steak is the leaner, healthier option for the meat-lover in your family.

Rice and Beans

2 tablespoons salted butter

2 shallots or 1 small red onion, finely chopped

2 garlic cloves, minced

1 cup white basmati rice

2 cups gluten-free chicken broth

1 15-ounce can black beans, drained and well rinsed

Grated zest and juice of 2 limes

2 bay leaves

¼ teaspoon salt

1. Prepare the steak: In a large stockpot, combine the flank steak, onions, carrots, celery, bay leaves, and black peppercorns. Add enough water to just cover the ingredients. Bring to a simmer and cook, partially covered, for about 1½ hours, or until the beef shreds easily when pressed with a fork.

2. When the meat is very tender, remove the pot from the heat and let the ingredients cool in the liquid for 20 minutes. Then remove the meat and strain the broth into a small bowl, discarding the vegetables and seasonings. Set the meat and the broth aside.

3. Make the sauce: Heat the olive oil in a large saucepan over medium heat, and add the chopped onion, bell pepper, and garlic. Sprinkle in the salt. Cook for 8 to 10 minutes, until the vegetables begin to soften. Then add the tomato paste, cumin, and oregano, and cook for 1 minute more, until the tomato paste becomes fragrant.

4. Stir in the reserved broth and simmer for 2 to 3 minutes, until the broth reduces slightly. Add the tomatoes and the shredded meat. Cook, uncovered, for 20 to 25 minutes, until the liquid has reduced by half.

5. While the meat is cooking in the sauce, prepare the rice and

Elisabeth Hasselbeck

beans: Heat a small saucepan over medium-high heat, and add the butter, shallots or red onion, and garlic. Cook for 2 to 3 minutes, until the shallots start to soften. Add the rice and cook, stirring often, for 1 minute, until the rice is completely coated in the butter.

6. Add the chicken broth, black beans, lime zest and juice, bay leaves, and salt. Stir to combine and bring to a boil. Then cover the pan, reduce the heat to low, and cook until the liquid has been absorbed and the rice is tender, 15 to 20 minutes. Remove and discard the bay leaves.

7. Serve the Ropa Vieja over the rice and beans.

Short Ribs with Parmesan Brussels Sprouts

When serving these ribs for a game-day gathering, I prep them in the morning so that they can simmer through the afternoon. One benefit to me is that the kitchen remains tidy while the ribs simmer, but the major benefit is that we all then get to eat them during the game! Be sure to set out extra napkins for sticky fingers; offer forks and serve these with your favorite side, like my Parmesan Brussels Sprouts or perhaps one of the mashed potato recipes on pages 118–120.

SERVES 8

When shopping for short ribs, the thicker the better since they shrink quite a bit during cooking.

4 to 5 pounds beef short ribs, cut into 3-inch pieces
½ teaspoon salt
¼ teaspoon freshly ground black pepper
1 tablespoon olive oil
1 yellow onion, finely chopped
3 garlic cloves, sliced
2 cups gluten-free beef broth
¼ cup packed gluten-free light brown sugar
1 tablespoon gluten-free Dijon mustard
2 tablespoons minced fresh flat-leaf parsley

1. Sprinkle the ribs with the salt and black pepper. Heat the olive oil in a Dutch oven or in a large, deep ovenproof skillet over high heat. Working in batches, add the ribs and cook, turning them once, until browned, 8 to 10 minutes. Transfer the ribs to a plate.

Elisabeth Hasselbeck

2. Reduce the heat to medium and add the onion and garlic to the skillet. Cook until softened, 2 to 3 minutes. Add 1 cup of the beef broth, scraping up any browned bits from the bottom of the skillet. Stir in the brown sugar and mustard. Return the ribs, with any accumulated juices, to the pot. Bring to a simmer and then cover partially. Cook until the meat is fork-tender, 2 to 2½ hours, adding more broth as needed so that the ribs are just covered with liquid as they cook.

3. Once the ribs are very tender, transfer them to a plate. Reduce any liquid remaining in the pot until you have about 1 cup of thick sauce. Pour the sauce over the ribs, and sprinkle the parsley on top as a garnish.

Parmesan Brussels Sprouts
Roasting Brussels sprouts is the way to go for great flavor and perfect texture. Boiling them can damage the sprouts' healthy cancer-fighting sulfur compounds and also leaves them limp.

SERVES 4

My kids actually like these. Need I say more?

1 tablespoon olive oil
1 pound Brussels sprouts, stem ends trimmed, cut in half
¼ teaspoon salt
¼ teaspoon freshly ground black pepper
½ cup shaved Parmesan cheese

1. Preheat the oven to 400°F.

2. Heat a large ovenproof skillet over medium-high heat. Add the olive oil and the Brussels sprouts, cut side down. Sprinkle the sprouts with the salt and black pepper. Cook, without turning, until they are a deep brown, 3 to 4 minutes.

3. Layer the shaved Parmesan over the sprouts, and slide the skillet into the oven. Bake for 3 to 4 minutes, until the Brussels sprouts are tender when pierced with a fork. Serve immediately.

Elisabeth Hasselbeck

Beef Stew

On winter nights that call for something hearty, beef stew is always at the top of the list in our home. This all-in-one dish makes this mom feel pretty great about getting a meal to the table that has it all—protein, veggies, and vitamins.

SERVES 4

¼ teaspoon salt

2 pounds lean cubed stew beef, trimmed of excess fat

¼ cup brown rice flour

2 teaspoons gluten-free sweet or hot Hungarian paprika

½ teaspoon freshly ground black pepper

2 tablespoons canola oil

1 large onion, sliced into thin rings

2 slices gluten-free bacon, chopped

4 garlic cloves, minced

2 tablespoons gluten-free tomato paste

½ cup dry white wine or red wine

4 cups gluten-free beef broth

4 carrots, cut into 1-inch chunks

1 large sweet potato, cubed

2 tablespoons chopped fresh flat-leaf parsley

Double-batching this one will provide another meal later in the week. Yes, it counts as homemade if you reheat something you made in the first place!

1. Sprinkle the salt over the meat. On a sheet of wax paper, mix the brown rice flour, paprika, and black pepper. Roll the beef cubes in the flour mixture to coat them. Set aside.

2. Heat 1 tablespoon of the canola oil in a large heavy-bottomed skillet over medium-high heat. Add the beef and cook, turning the pieces once or twice, until they are golden, 5 to 7 minutes. Transfer the beef to a plate.

3. Add the remaining 1 tablespoon canola oil to the skillet, and add the onion, bacon, and garlic. Cook for 4 to 5 minutes, until the onion begins to soften and brown. Then reduce the heat to low, add the tomato paste, and cook for 1 minute, stirring well. Add the wine and bring to a simmer.

4. Return all the meat and any accumulated juices to the skillet. Add the beef broth, scraping up any browned bits and pieces from the bottom of the pan. Bring the stew to a steady simmer (you may need to raise the heat to medium). Cover, and simmer until the meat is fork-tender, 2 to 2½ hours.

5. Add the carrots and sweet potato to the stew and cook for 30 minutes, until the carrots are tender. Spoon into warmed soup plates, garnish with the parsley, and serve.

Beef Stroganoff

Here's another perfect wintertime dish—rich, filling, warm, and comforting. It might taste as if it has been simmering for hours, but it cooks in under 20 minutes!

SERVES 4

2 pounds boneless top sirloin, cut into thin strips about 1 inch wide and 2 inches long

½ teaspoon salt

¼ teaspoon freshly ground black pepper

2 tablespoons olive oil

2 tablespoons salted butter

1 pound cremini or white button mushrooms, sliced

1 large white onion, finely chopped

1 tablespoon gluten-free tomato paste

2 tablespoons amaranth or brown rice flour

2 cups gluten-free beef broth

½ cup gluten-free light sour cream

2 teaspoons gluten-free Dijon mustard

¼ cup fresh flat-leaf parsley leaves, thinly sliced or chopped

1. Sprinkle the beef strips with the salt and black pepper. Heat a large skillet over high heat. When the skillet is hot, add 1 tablespoon of the olive oil and half of the beef. Cook, turning the strips once or twice, for about 2 minutes, until they start to brown but are still pink in spots. Transfer the beef to a bowl. Repeat with the remaining tablespoon of olive oil and the remaining beef. Add it to the bowl.

2. In the same skillet over medium heat, melt the butter. Add the mushrooms and onion, and cook, stirring occasionally, for 4 to 5 minutes.

3. Add the tomato paste and stir until it coats the onion and mushrooms, about 1 minute. Then sprinkle the amaranth or brown rice flour over the vegetables and stir to incorporate. Raise the heat to high, add the beef broth, and bring to a boil, stirring with a wooden spoon to scrape up the browned bits clinging to the bottom and sides of the skillet. Reduce the heat to low. Return the meat and any accumulated juices to the skillet and cook just until the beef is heated through, about 2 minutes.

4. Scoop out ½ cup of the sauce and place it in a small bowl. Whisk in the sour cream and the mustard. Then pour the mixture into the skillet and stir gently to incorporate. Garnish with the parsley and serve immediately.

Elisabeth Hasselbeck

Beef Fajitas with Peppers and Onions

Full of flavor and sizzle, fajitas make beef more fun! They are even more fun when g-free-ers can eat them too. Your family will lobby to have them at least once a week.

SERVES 4

1 pound beef round, sliced into stir-fry strips

1 teaspoon gluten-free mild chili powder

½ teaspoon gluten-free ground cumin

½ teaspoon dried oregano

½ teaspoon cornstarch

½ teaspoon salt

¼ teaspoon freshly ground black pepper

⅛ teaspoon gluten-free garlic powder

⅛ teaspoon gluten-free onion powder

2 tablespoons olive oil

1 red bell pepper, seeded and sliced into ¼-inch-thick rings

1 green bell pepper, seeded and sliced into ¼-inch-thick rings

1 large red onion, sliced into ¼-inch-thick rings

12 gluten-free corn tortillas, warmed

6 ounces Monterey Jack cheese, grated

1 15-ounce jar gluten-free tomato salsa, for serving (optional)

To mix things up, and for other colors and textures, try using sliced mushrooms, small broccoli florets, or fresh corn kernels in place of the peppers.

1. Spread the beef strips out on a sheet of wax paper, and sprinkle them with the chili powder, cumin, oregano, cornstarch, salt, black pepper, garlic powder, and onion powder.

2. Heat a large skillet over medium-high heat and add 1 tablespoon of the olive oil and the beef. Cook, turning often, until the outside is browned but the meat is still slightly pink on the inside, 3 to 4 minutes. Transfer the meat to a plate.

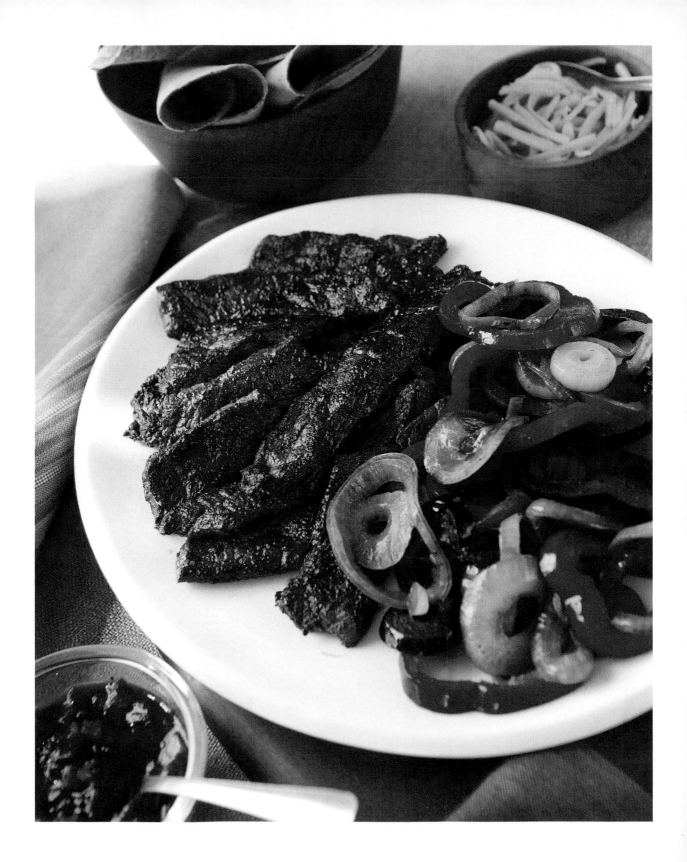

3. Add the remaining 1 tablespoon olive oil, the red and green bell peppers, and the onion to the skillet. Cook, stirring often, for 3 to 4 minutes, until the onion and peppers are soft.

4. Serve the meat immediately. To assemble the fajitas, divide the beef among the tortillas, top with the vegetables and the cheese, and roll up the tortillas. Serve with salsa on the side, if desired.

Super Mimi's Grilled Flank Steak

Tim's grandmother, who has earned the title "Super Mimi," is just that: a most incredible woman in every way. A mother to twelve fun, engaging, and kind children of her own, she is always organizing games for her sixty-three (and counting) grandchildren and great-grandchildren.

Super Mimi really knows her meat. She was the first female butcher in Cincinnati and a lefty at that. You should see her carve! She also makes the tastiest flank steak around—and I hope I do the g-free version justice!

SERVES 8

1 large flank steak (about 2 pounds)
½ cup gluten-free low-sodium soy sauce
½ cup gluten-free Worcestershire sauce
½ teaspoon gluten-free mustard powder, or to taste
Juice of 1 lemon

1. Using a sharp paring knife, score the flank steak on both sides. Pat both sides dry with a paper towel. Place the soy sauce, Worcestershire sauce, mustard powder, and lemon juice in a large zipper-lock bag. Add the flank steak and flip to coat it in the marinade. Marinate for 1 whole day (24 hours), turning the bag so that both sides of the steak are covered in the marinade.

2. Heat a large grill pan over high heat. Remove the flank steak from the marinade and pat it dry with paper towels. Place the

Elisabeth Hasselbeck

flank steak on the grill pan and cook, turning it over once or twice, 10 to 12 minutes for medium-rare and 12 to 14 minutes for medium.

3. Transfer the steak to a cutting board and let it rest for 5 minutes to allow the juices to redistribute, then thinly slice the flank steak, and serve.

Here's a helpful hint for getting the most juice that you can from a lemon: microwave the whole lemon for a quick two seconds before you slice it open to squeeze!

Chimichurri Flank Steak and Grilled Asparagus

Are you a garlic-lover? If so, dig in to this recipe! Chimichurri is a garlicky green sauce that comes from the ranching culture in Argentina. You can also use this fragrant sauce as a marinade for chicken or shrimp.

SERVES 4

Chimichurri Sauce
1½ cups firmly packed fresh flat-leaf parsley leaves
2 tablespoons fresh oregano leaves
4 garlic cloves, quartered
1 tablespoon red wine vinegar
1 teaspoon salt
¼ teaspoon freshly ground black pepper
¼ teaspoon gluten-free red pepper flakes
½ cup extra-virgin olive oil

1 large flank steak (about 2 pounds)
1 pound asparagus spears, trimmed

1. Prepare the chimichurri sauce: Place the parsley, oregano, garlic, vinegar, salt, black pepper, and red pepper flakes in a food processor. Process until finely chopped. With the motor running, drizzle in the olive oil until it's completely incorporated. Set aside.

2. Preheat a large barbecue grill.

3. Brush a tablespoon of the chimichurri sauce over each side of the flank steak. Grill the steak on one side, without moving it,

Elisabeth Hasselbeck

for 4 minutes. Turn it over and grill for 4 to 6 minutes on the other side for medium-rare, or until done to your liking.

4. Transfer the steak to a carving board, cover it loosely with aluminum foil, and let it rest for 5 minutes.

5. While the steak is resting, grill the asparagus, turning the spears often, until they are fork-tender, 5 minutes.

6. Cut the steak diagonally across the grain into ¼-inch-thick slices. Transfer the meat and the asparagus to a large platter, and top with 2 generous spoonfuls of the chimichurri. Pass the remaining sauce at the table.

Stuffed Cabbage

My dad is of Polish descent and he has long been making dishes from that heritage. Serve this saucy meal with mashed potatoes (see page 118–120) or buttered g-free noodles.

SERVES 10 (MAKES ABOUT 20 STUFFED CABBAGE ROLLS)

1 1-pound head of Savoy or green cabbage

1 pound ground lean beef

1 pound ground pork

2 cups carrots, grated

1 small onion, finely chopped or grated

½ cup gluten-free brown rice, cooked according to the package instructions

¼ cup chopped fresh flat-leaf parsley

1 teaspoon salt

½ teaspoon gluten-free paprika

¼ teaspoon freshly ground black pepper

1 teaspoon olive oil

¼ cup gluten-free tomato paste

2 cups gluten-free beef broth

1 28-ounce can diced tomatoes, with juices

1. Fill a large stockpot half full with water, and bring it to a boil. Using a paring knife, cut out and discard the core of the cabbage. Submerge the cabbage, core side up, in the boiling water. Using a fork or tongs, begin to peel the outer leaves off the cabbage as soon as they become soft. Continue to peel the leaves off, transferring them to a bowl. Once you can no longer peel the leaves off easily, remove the remaining center of the cabbage from

The cancer-fighting properties of cabbage in this one can't be beat.

Elisabeth Hasselbeck

the stockpot and discard the cooking water. Coarsely chop the center of the cabbage, and set it aside separately.

2. In a large bowl, combine the ground beef, ground pork, carrots, onion, cooked brown rice, parsley, salt, paprika, and black pepper. Mix well. Using a paring knife, trim any hard spines from the cabbage leaves so they will fold easily. Place about ¼ cup of the meat mixture on the inside of a cabbage leaf where it was attached to the core. Fold the bottom of the leaf over the filling and fold the sides over. Roll the cabbage leaf up. Repeat until you have used all the filling.

3. In the same stockpot you used for cooking the cabbage, heat the olive oil over medium heat. Add the tomato paste and cook for 1 minute, until it starts to brown. Then add the beef broth and whisk to combine. Tuck the stuffed cabbage rolls, seam side down, into the pot, and scatter the chopped cabbage over them. Pour the diced tomatoes over the chopped cabbage, place the pot over medium-low heat, and cover. Cook for 40 to 45 minutes, until the sauce has reduced by one third, the cabbage is tender, and the meat is cooked through. Serve immediately.

Stuffed "Perfetto" Peppers

Just like my Mama, my mom and my aunt Mickey have always made these perfetto stuffed peppers. If you want to make them leaner, swap the ground pork for ground turkey (but trust me on this one: in this case, it is so worth it to keep the pork!).

SERVES 8

5 ounces baby spinach
½ pound ground sirloin
½ pound ground pork
1 10-ounce container white button mushrooms, chopped
1 teaspoon salt
4 red, yellow, orange, or green bell peppers
1 tablespoon olive oil
1 medium, bone-in pork chop (about ¼ pound)
2 garlic cloves, thinly sliced
2 28-ounce cans diced tomatoes, with juices
¼ cup gluten-free tomato paste
1 fresh basil sprig

1. Heat a large skillet over high heat. Add the spinach and 2 tablespoons of water. Cook for about 30 seconds or until the spinach wilts. Transfer the spinach to a cutting board, and when it is cool enough to handle, chop it fine. Place the chopped spinach in a large bowl and add the ground sirloin, ground pork, mushrooms, and salt. Mix well with your fingers until the spinach is evenly distributed.

2. Use a small paring knife to cut around the stems of the bell peppers, leaving a ½-inch margin. Pull out the seeds and the

Elisabeth Hasselbeck

white membrane that holds the seeds. Rinse out the inside of the peppers with cold running water. Drain, and then stuff the peppers with the meat mixture.

3. Heat a large stockpot over medium-high heat. Add the olive oil and the pork chop. Cook for 3 to 4 minutes until the chop begins to brown, turning the pork chop once or twice. Add the garlic and cook for 1 minute, until it is fragrant. Stand the pork chop up against the inside of the pot, and then carefully add the peppers to the pot, filling side up.

4. Pour in the tomatoes along with their juices, and add the tomato paste, basil sprig, and ½ cup of water. Bring to a steady simmer; then reduce the heat to medium-low. Cover partially and cook for 45 minutes to 1 hour. Remove and discard the basil sprig. Serve immediately.

Tacos with Salsa Verde

Everyone looks forward to weekly taco night at our house. Tacos allow the kids a fun way to be helpful—putting cheese in the bowl, chopping tomatoes, shredding lettuce. Their reward is building their own taco in a taco shell or a tortilla and by choosing their own toppings, and my reward is watching them enjoy dinner, complaint-free!

SERVES 4

There are lots of store-bought g-free options for taco mixes, but g-free doesn't mean chemical- or additive-free or low-calorie. This make-your-own seasoning mix recipe offers a solution that will have you saying Olé!

1 tablespoon olive oil

1 pound ground sirloin

2 teaspoons cornstarch

2 teaspoons gluten-free mild chili powder

1 teaspoon gluten-free ground cumin

½ teaspoon salt

¼ teaspoon freshly ground black pepper, or to taste

1 cup gluten-free beef broth

4 5-inch gluten-free corn tortillas

4 gluten-free taco shells

1 cup shredded pepper Jack, cheddar, or Monterey Jack cheese

1 avocado, pitted, peeled, and thinly sliced

2 cups thinly sliced romaine lettuce leaves

2 large tomatoes, diced

¼ red onion, minced

1. Heat a large skillet over high heat. Add the olive oil and the ground sirloin. Cook the meat for 1 minute without stirring. Then cook for 3 to 4 minutes longer, stirring occasionally, until most of the meat is brown. Sprinkle the cornstarch, chili powder, cumin, salt, and black pepper over the meat. Add the beef broth

Elisabeth Hasselbeck

and cook for 8 to 10 minutes, until a thick sauce has formed and the beef is tender.

2. Meanwhile, warm the tortillas and the taco shells as directed on their packaging.

3. Stuff the tortillas and taco shells with the meat, and sprinkle with the cheese. Top with your choice of avocado, lettuce, tomatoes, and/or onion, and serve immediately.

Salsa Verde *Take your tacos up a gourmet notch while adding a spicy kick with this easy-to-make salsa. Tomatillos are part of the gooseberry family and have similar papery husks. You can find them in gourmet groceries and in Latin markets.*

MAKES 2 CUPS

1 pound tomatillos (about 8 medium), husks removed and discarded
½ red onion, skin intact
2 jalapeños
¼ cup fresh cilantro leaves
Juice of 1 large lime
1 teaspoon fresh oregano leaves, chopped
½ teaspoon salt

Don't bite into a raw tomatillo. Boiling changes their taste and texture for the better.

1. Bring a large saucepan of water to a boil. With a sharp paring knife, cut a large "x" on the bottom of each tomatillo. Place the tomatillos in the boiling water and cook for 3 to 4 minutes, until the skins soften but the tomatillos do not become mushy. Remove from the hot water and rinse with cold water. Drain and set aside.

2. Heat a small skillet over high heat for 1 minute. Add the red onion and the jalapeños. Roast for 4 to 5 minutes, turning them occasionally with tongs, until the skin of the onion and jalapeños begins to blacken.

3. Remove the papery skin from the onion half and cut the onion into quarters. Remove the seeds and stems from the jalapeños. Place the jalapeños and the onion quarters in a food processor.

4. Peel off and discard the tomatillo skins, and add the tomatillos to the food processor. Add the cilantro, lime juice, oregano, and salt, and process until smooth.

Black Bean Soup

This winter soup is packed with flavor, without packing in the calories. To make it an even heartier bowlful, add chopped cooked chicken or steak. To accommodate a vegetarian diet, swap out the chicken broth for gluten-free vegetable broth.

SERVES 8

2 tablespoons olive oil
1 small red onion, chopped
1 red or orange bell pepper, seeded and chopped
¼ cup packed fresh cilantro leaves
1 jalapeño, seeded and minced
2 garlic cloves, minced
½ teaspoon salt
1 quart gluten-free chicken broth
2 15-ounce cans black beans, drained and well rinsed
1 15-ounce can diced tomatoes, with juices
1 cup sour cream, for serving

1. Heat a large stockpot over medium-high heat. Add the olive oil, onion, bell pepper, cilantro, jalapeño, garlic, and salt. Cook, stirring occasionally, for 3 to 4 minutes, as the onion and peppers soften.

2. Add the chicken broth, beans, and diced tomatoes, and raise the heat to high. As soon as the soup comes to a boil, reduce the heat to low and simmer, uncovered, for 25 to 30 minutes, until the liquid has decreased by one third. Serve immediately, with the sour cream alongside.

Bistro Burgers

Burgers are a classic hit on any night, but with a little gluten-free seasoning and your own choice of toppings, you can make them just a tad gourmet. Keep the meal a hands-on affair by serving sides like sweet potato chips and fun crisp veggies.

SERVES 8

My personal favorite is a burger with gluten-free barbecue sauce and a slice of cheddar cheese.

1 pound 90% lean ground beef

1 pound 85% lean ground beef

6 tablespoons gluten-free Worcestershire sauce or gluten-free ketchup

2 tablespoons salt

¼ teaspoon freshly ground black pepper

8 slices cheddar or Swiss cheese (optional)

8 gluten-free hamburger buns, split

2 tablespoons gluten-free barbecue sauce, per burger

8 slices tomato (about 2 medium tomatoes; optional)

8 slices sweet white onion, such as Vidalia (optional)

8 pieces romaine lettuce (optional)

1. Prepare a charcoal or gas grill for direct grilling over medium-high heat.

2. In a large bowl, combine both types of beef, the Worcestershire sauce or ketchup, and the salt and black pepper. Form the mixture into 8 patties, each ¾ inch thick.

3. Grill the hamburgers directly over medium-high heat, turning them once, for 3 to 5 minutes per side. Check for doneness by testing with an instant-read thermometer (it should reach 160°F) or by using a paring knife to check for pinkness inside (there should be no translucent red inside). If you are making cheese-burgers, place a slice of cheese on top of each hamburger during the last 3 minutes of cooking.

4. Toast the hamburger buns, cut side down, on the grill. Serve the hamburgers immediately on the buns, with the barbecue sauce, tomato, onion, and lettuce, if using.

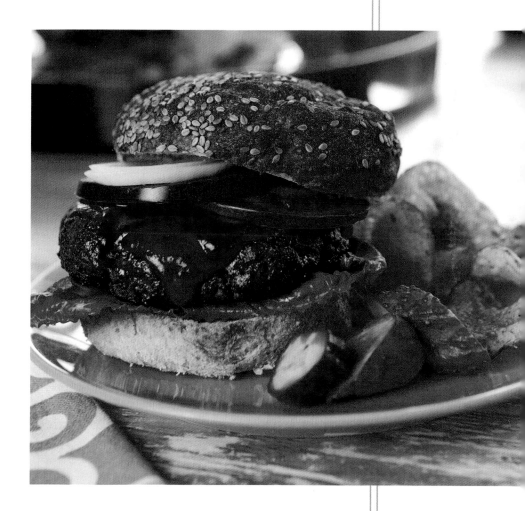

Sunday Roast with Carrots and Potatoes

Pair this with one of my mashed potato recipes (pages 118–120) and you'll be crowned queen or king of your family feast. Be sure to trim the fat well from your roast before searing it, to keep the sauce from becoming too oily.

SERVES 8

1 yellow onion, finely chopped
4 carrots, finely chopped
1 pound red-skinned potatoes, cut into ½-inch pieces
2 cups gluten-free beef broth
3 tablespoons gluten-free tomato paste
4 garlic cloves, crushed
3 fresh thyme sprigs, or 1 large fresh rosemary sprig
1 bay leaf
1 beef rump roast (3 to 4 pounds)
1 teaspoon salt
¼ teaspoon freshly ground black pepper
2 tablespoons brown rice flour
2 tablespoons millet flour
1 tablespoon olive oil

1. Put the onion, carrots, potatoes, beef broth, tomato paste, garlic, thyme or rosemary, and bay leaf in a slow-cooker and stir to combine.

2. Season the roast with the salt and black pepper. Put the brown rice flour and the millet flour in a large bowl, and stir them together. Add the roast and turn to coat it evenly.

Elisabeth Hasselbeck

3. In a large sauté pan over medium-high heat, warm the olive oil until it is nearly smoking. Add the roast and brown it on all sides, 3 to 4 minutes total. Transfer the roast to the slow-cooker, cover, and cook on the high setting for 6 hours.

4. Transfer the roast to a carving board, cover it loosely with aluminum foil, and let it rest for 5 minutes. Then slice the meat and arrange it on a warmed platter. Remove and discard the bay leaf and herb sprigs, and serve the vegetables and sauce alongside the meat.

Boneless Pork Ribs

This meal is so easy and flavorful that I almost feel guilty when people think I spent hours in the kitchen over it! This is the recipe that I turn to when I need a meal that can satisfy any appetite. Try pairing them with my delicious baked bean recipe that follows.

SERVES 8

2 tablespoons canola oil

2 pounds boneless pork ribs

1 large sweet onion, such as Vidalia or Walla Walla

2 small jalapeños or 1 green bell pepper, seeded and chopped

2 tablespoons gluten-free light brown sugar

¼ teaspoon freshly ground black pepper

1 18-ounce jar (2¼ cups) gluten-free barbecue sauce

1. Heat a large stockpot over medium-high heat and add the canola oil. Add the pork ribs and brown for 3 to 4 minutes, turning them once. Transfer the ribs to a plate.

2. Add the onion, jalapeños or bell pepper, brown sugar, and black pepper to the stockpot. Cook over medium heat, stirring often, until the onion and peppers start to soften, 3 to 4 minutes.

3. Return the pork ribs along with the barbecue sauce to the stockpot and reduce the heat to a slow simmer. Cover, and cook over low heat for 20 to 25 minutes, until the ribs are tender. Serve immediately.

Elisabeth Hasselbeck

Baked Beans

To round out your al fresco fiesta, summer barbecue, or family reunion, be sure to try this American potluck classic. Full of fiber and flavor, this dish does double duty: it's both healthy and hearty.

SERVES 8

1 tablespoon canola or olive oil
1 large yellow onion, finely chopped
2 carrots, finely grated
1 2-ounce gluten-free slice slab bacon or salt pork, chopped
2 15-ounce cans pinto beans, drained and well rinsed
½ cup pure maple syrup
1 tablespoon gluten-free tomato paste
¼ cup firmly packed gluten-free dark brown sugar
2 teaspoons apple cider vinegar or gluten-free rice vinegar
½ teaspoon salt

1. Preheat the oven to 325°F.

2. Heat a medium Dutch oven or heavy-bottomed ovenproof saucepan over medium heat. Add the canola or olive oil, onion, carrots, and bacon or salt pork, and reduce the heat to medium-low. Cook, stirring occasionally, until the vegetables are well browned and softened, about 20 minutes. Remove the pan from the heat. Add the beans, maple syrup, tomato paste, brown sugar, vinegar, and salt, and stir to combine.

3. Transfer the pan to the oven and bake, uncovered, until a golden crust forms and the beans are very tender, 20 to 25 minutes. Let the beans cool for 5 minutes, and then serve.

Pork Chop Dinner with Caramelized Onions, Apples, and Green Beans

This is one meal that will give you bragging rights to be called Queen of the Kitchen! For kids, you might want to substitute applesauce for the onion and apple mixture, but the grown-up version here is a home run! Some nights, I'll make extra caramelized onions and apples to serve on grilled chicken or burgers later in the week. Once you serve it up, you will understand why.

SERVES 4

3 tablespoons canola or olive oil

1 large sweet onion, such as Walla Walla or Vidalia, cut into rings

2 tablespoons firmly packed gluten-free light brown sugar

¾ teaspoon salt

2 apples, such as Golden Delicious or Gala, cored and thinly sliced

2 tablespoons apple cider vinegar

4 bone-in pork chops, each about ¾ inch thick (about 2 pounds total), trimmed of excess fat

¼ teaspoon freshly ground black pepper

1 pound green beans, trimmed

1 pound baby carrots

1 tablespoon salted butter

1. Heat a large skillet over high heat. Add 2 tablespoons of the canola or olive oil and the onion, brown sugar, and ¼ teaspoon of the salt. Reduce the heat to medium-low and cook for 10 to 15 minutes, stirring often, until the onion is golden brown. If the

onion starts to brown too quickly or to stick, add a few table-spoons of water and continue cooking.

2. Add the apple slices to the onion and cook, turning the apples often, for 2 to 3 minutes. Add the vinegar and cook for 1 minute more, until the apples are soft. Set aside.

3. Preheat the oven to 400°F.

4. Sprinkle the pork chops with the remaining ¼ teaspoon salt and the black pepper. Heat another large skillet over high heat. Remove the skillet from heat and coat with cooking spray. Return it to the heat, and add the pork chops. Cook for 4 to 5 minutes, turning once. Slide the skillet into the oven and bake the pork chops for 12 to 15 minutes, until cooked through. Top with the onion and apple mixture, cover, and set aside.

5. Meanwhile, heat a large skillet over high heat. Add the remaining 1 tablespoon canola or olive oil and remaining salt. Add the green beans and carrots and cook for 1 to 2 minutes, tossing until the vegetables are coated in the oil. Add ½ cup of water, cover the skillet, and cook for 3 to 4 minutes, or until the vegetables are tender. Remove from the heat and add the butter. Toss to coat, and serve immediately with the pork chops.

Pulled Pork

The first time I served this to a large crowd, it turned out to be the life of the party! Now it's my go-to recipe for most casual gatherings. For anyone on a paleo- or low-carb diet, you can serve the pork in lettuce leaves (butter lettuce is best) instead of buns.

MAKES 10 SANDWICHES

Nonstick cooking spray
1 5-pound pork loin end roast, well trimmed of fat
½ teaspoon sea salt
2 teaspoons olive oil
2 large Vidalia onions, cut into 1-inch-thick slices
4 garlic cloves, crushed
1 cup dry white wine
1 18-ounce jar gluten-free barbecue sauce
¼ cup gluten-free light brown sugar
1 canned gluten-free chipotle en adobo, plus 1 tablespoon adobo sauce
10 gluten-free hamburger buns; or 10 gluten-free tortillas, warmed

1. Grease a large skillet with a generous layer of cooking spray, and heat it over high heat.

2. Sprinkle both sides of the pork roast with the sea salt, place it in the skillet, and cook, turning it occasionally, until it is browned on all sides, 8 to 10 minutes. Transfer the roast to a slow-cooker on the high setting, or to a stockpot set over low heat.

3. Place the olive oil and onions in the same skillet. Reduce the heat to medium-low and cook, stirring occasionally, until the onions begin to soften, 8 to 10 minutes. Add a tablespoon of water

Elisabeth Hasselbeck

if they begin to stick. Add the garlic and cook for 2 minutes, or until it becomes fragrant.

4. Transfer the onions and garlic to the slow-cooker or stockpot. Pour the wine into the skillet and scrape up any brown bits from the bottom of the pan. Add the wine mixture to the cooker or stockpot, and then add the barbecue sauce, brown sugar, and chipotle with the adobo sauce. Cover, and cook in the slow-cooker for 6 to 8 hours on high, or simmer in the stockpot over low heat for 3½ to 4 hours, until the meat is tender and beginning to break apart.

5. Break up the meat with a fork and stir it back into the sauce. Serve on the hamburger buns or tortillas.

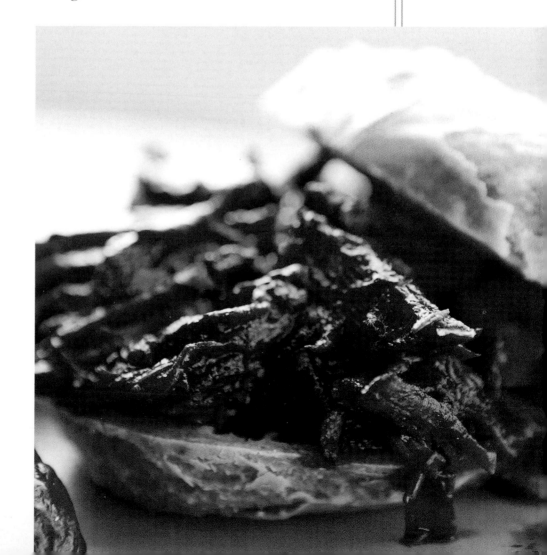

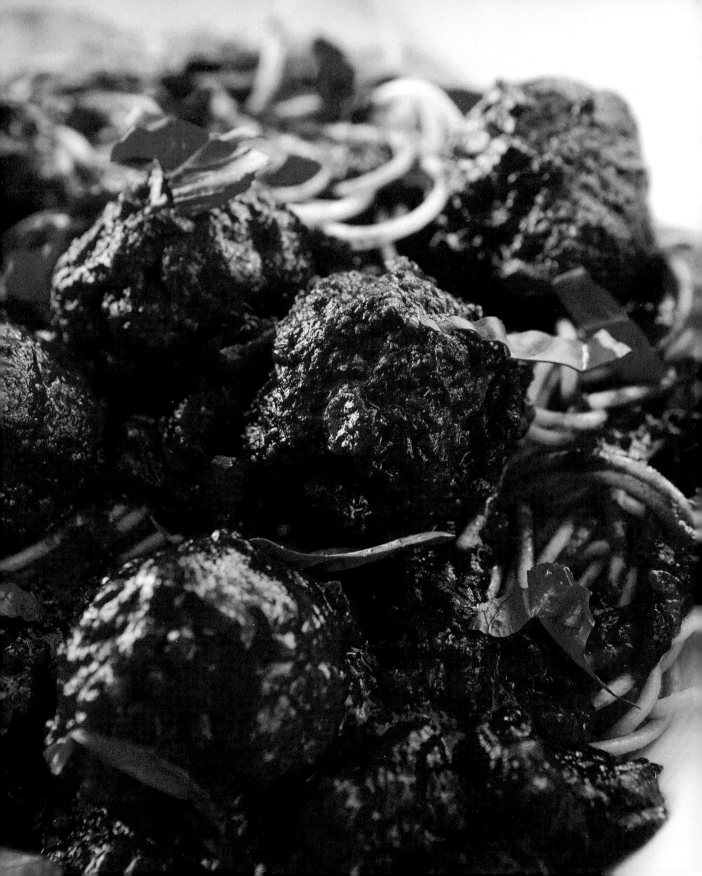

Mama's Spaghetti and Meatballs

I mentioned the significance of this meal to me in this book's introduction: it was part of my childhood and was one of the things I missed most when I initially went g-free. Now, thanks to the great work of my mom, who translated my grandmother's recipe from glutenous to g-free, you too can enjoy it. As we say in my family, "Buono, buono!"

SERVES 10 (MAKES ABOUT 2 CUPS OF SAUCE AND 30 MEATBALLS)

Meatballs

½ cup gluten-free hominy grits or coarse cornmeal, or crumbs from
   2 slices gluten-free bread
1 ½ pounds ground chuck
1 egg, beaten lightly
1 garlic clove, minced
2 tablespoons chopped fresh flat-leaf parsley
2 tablespoons grated Romano or Parmesan cheese
1 teaspoon salt
¼ teaspoon freshly ground black pepper
1 tablespoon light olive oil or canola oil, or more if needed

Tomato and Meat Sauce

1 pound gluten-free sweet or hot Italian sausage
3 tablespoons olive oil
1 small onion, minced in a food processor
3 28-ounce cans crushed tomatoes
1 teaspoon granulated sugar
1 teaspoon salt

I often use a slow-cooker to make this sauce. I brown the sausage and onion in a large skillet first, and am always sure to scrape up all the brown bits from the pan (using a little water to help the process) when adding it all to the cooker.

½ teaspoon freshly ground black pepper

3 or 4 fresh basil leaves

2 pounds dried spaghetti

1. Prepare the meatballs: In a small bowl, combine 1½ table-spoons of water with the grits, cornmeal, or bread crumbs. Mix to moisten; the grits/cornmeal/crumbs should be damp but not wet. Set aside.

2. Place the ground chuck in a large bowl. Add the egg, garlic, parsley, grated Romano or Parmesan, salt, and black pepper, and mix with a wooden spoon. Add the moistened grits/cornmeal/crumbs and mix, first with the spoon and then with your hands, just until the ingredients are combined.

3. Shape the meat mixture into meatballs about the size of golf balls.

4. Heat a large skillet over medium-high heat, and add the olive or canola oil. Working in batches so as not to crowd the skillet, and adding more oil as needed, cook the meatballs until they are browned, about 1 to 2 minutes. As they are cooked, transfer the meatballs to a plate and set aside for use in the tomato sauce, or cover and refrigerate or freeze until you are ready to make the sauce. The meatballs will keep in the refrigerator for up to 5 days and in the freezer for up to 3 months.

5. Prepare the sauce: Cut the sausage into 2-inch pieces. Heat the olive oil in a Dutch oven or other large, heavy pot, and brown the sausage on all sides in the oil. Add the minced onion and cook it with the sausage until the onion is soft and light brown, about 4 to 5 minutes.

6. Add 1 can of the crushed tomatoes to the pot. Fill the can about one-quarter full with water, swish it around to rinse out the can, and pour the water into the pot. Stir, scraping up the brown

bits from the bottom of the pot. Add the remaining 2 cans of tomatoes, rinsing each can with ¼ can of water as before and adding the water to the pot. Add the sugar, salt, black pepper, and basil leaves, and stir to mix. Add the meatballs and stir.

7. Bring the sauce to a boil over medium-high heat, stirring occasionally; then lower the heat to a slow simmer. Simmer the sauce for 30 minutes, or longer if desired. (I like to simmer the sauce until I see that the oil has risen to the top.) Stir occasionally to prevent sticking.

8. When you are ready to serve, bring a large pot of salted water to a boil. Add the spaghetti and cook according to the package directions. Then drain, and serve topped with the pasta sauce.

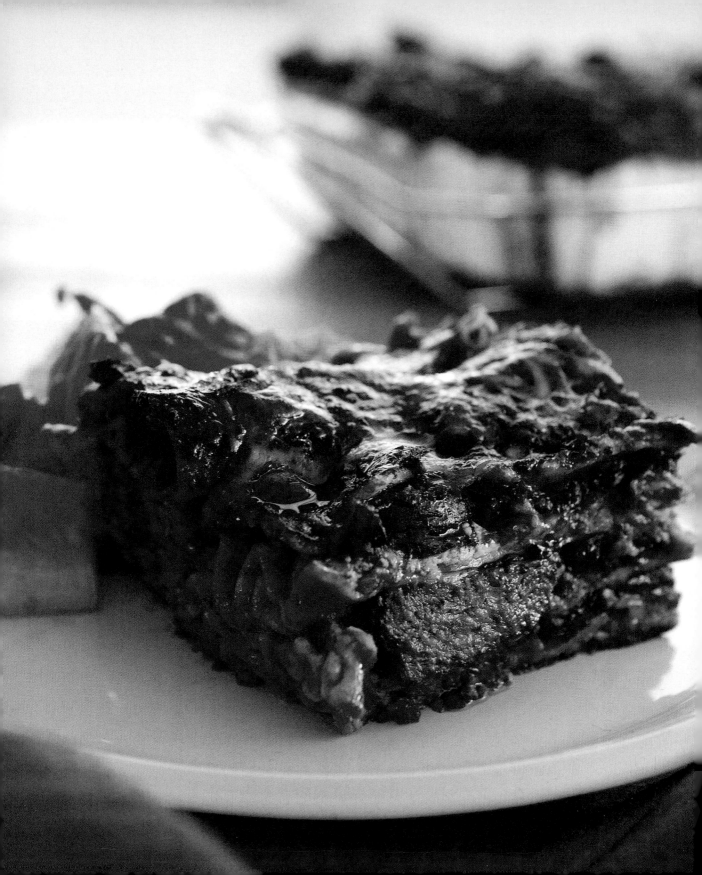

Lasagna

Are you hosting a big family dinner anytime soon? Well, here's a chance to take the pressure off: make it Italian and make it the night before. Preparing the lasagna ahead also gives it time to "set," as my Mama would say, making the pieces easier to cut.

SERVES 12

1 pound ricotta cheese

1 egg, lightly beaten

¼ cup chopped fresh flat-leaf parsley

½ cup gluten-free hominy grits, coarse cornmeal, or gluten-free rice crumbs

1½ teaspoons salt

½ teaspoon freshly ground black pepper

Pinch of gluten-free ground cinnamon (optional)

3 to 4 cups Tomato and Meat Sauce (see page 161)

¾ to 1 pound shredded low-moisture mozzarella; or ¾- to 1-pound ball of low-moisture mozzarella, cut into ½-inch cubes

¾ cup grated Romano or Parmesan cheese

1 tablespoon olive or canola oil

1½ pounds gluten-free lasagna noodles

Grated Romano or Parmesan cheese, for serving (optional)

Warmed Pasta Sauce (page 161), without the sausage and meatballs, for serving (optional)

> To reheat any leftover lasagna, just cover the pan, pop it into a preheated 200°F oven, and bake for 30 minutes.

1. Preheat the oven to 375°F.

2. In a large bowl, mix together the ricotta, egg, parsley, grits/cornmeal/crumbs, ½ teaspoon of the salt, the black pepper, and the cinnamon if using. Set aside. (If you are using gluten-free rice crumbs, which are harder than cornmeal, add ¼ cup of water and allow the rice crumbs to soften for several minutes.)

3. Remove half of the meatballs and half of the sausage pieces from the Tomato and Meat Sauce. Set the pasta sauce aside. Slice the meatballs and the sausage, and set aside.

4. Set aside and reserve (for topping the lasagna) 2 tablespoons of the mozzarella (about 4 cubes if you are using fresh mozzarella) and 2 tablespoons of the grated Romano or Parmesan, as well as about ½ cup of the pasta sauce.

5. Add the remaining 1 teaspoon salt and the olive or canola oil to a large pot of water (the oil will prevent the noodles from sticking), and bring the water to a boil. Add the lasagna noodles and cook for 6 to 7 minutes. (The noodles should be harder than al dente because they will continue to cook when baked.) Drain the noodles in a colander.

6. While the noodles are cooking, spoon about ½ cup of the pasta sauce over the bottom of a lasagna pan or a 9 × 13-inch baking dish.

7. Arrange a layer of cooked lasagna noodles over the sauce in the lasagna pan. By the spoonful, drop one third of the ricotta mixture over the layer of noodles, and then spread the ricotta out into an even layer. Scatter one third of the sliced meatballs and sausage over the ricotta. Sprinkle one third of the shredded or cubed mozzarella as the next layer. Next, spread about ⅓ cup of the pasta sauce over the mozzarella, and sprinkle one third of the grated cheese over the sauce.

8. Repeat the layers of cooked lasagna noodles, ricotta, meatballs and sausage, mozzarella, pasta sauce, and grated cheese. Then repeat the layers one more time.

9. Cover the top with a layer of cooked lasagna noodles. Spoon a thin layer of pasta sauce over the noodles, making sure it reaches the corners. Sprinkle the reserved mozzarella and then the re-

Elisabeth Hasselbeck

served grated cheese over the sauce. Cover the pan with aluminum foil.

10. Bake the lasagna until the corners are bubbling, 30 to 40 minutes. Then remove the foil and bake uncovered for another 7 to 10 minutes, until brown on top.

11. Remove the baked lasagna from the oven, cover it with foil, and let it stand for 10 minutes before cutting and serving.

12. Cut the lasagna into squares and serve with extra grated cheese and warm tomato sauce on the side, if desired.

Baked Penne

The pasta-lovers in your life are going to be spoiled by this recipe—it tastes just like the one that my Mama put on the table every weekend. The aroma brings me back to the days of "sneaking" a bite before it even got to the table. My grandmother would just smile at me as though to say, "I won't tell a soul. I am just so happy you like it!"

SERVES 12

3 to 4 cups Tomato and Meat Sauce (see page 161)
1 teaspoon salt
1 pound gluten-free penne or ziti
¾ pound low-moisture mozzarella, cut into ½-inch cubes or shredded
¾ cup grated Romano or Parmesan cheese
Grated Romano or Parmesan cheese, for serving (optional)
Warmed Pasta Sauce (page 161), without the sausage and meatballs, for
    serving (optional)

1. Preheat the oven to 375°F.

2. Remove half of the meatballs and half of the sausage pieces from the Tomato and Meat Sauce. Set the pasta sauce aside. Slice the meatballs and sausage, and set them aside.

3. Add the salt to a large pot of water and bring the water to a boil. Add the penne or ziti and cook for 6 to 7 minutes. (The pasta should be harder than al dente because it will continue to cook when baked.) Drain the pasta and return it to the pot.

4. Add about 2 cups of the pasta sauce to the pot and mix with a wooden spoon until the sauce is evenly distributed. Reserving 2 tablespoons of each cheese for the topping, add the mozzarella and the grated cheese to the pasta, and mix with the spoon. Then,

Elisabeth Hasselbeck

reserving ⅓ cup of each for the topping, add the slices of meatballs and sausage. Mix gently with the wooden spoon.

5. Spoon about ½ cup of the pasta sauce over the bottom of a lasagna pan or a 9 × 13-inch baking dish. Spoon the pasta mixture over the sauce, spreading it out evenly. Sprinkle the reserved mozzarella, and then the reserved grated cheese, on top, and cover the pan with aluminum foil.

6. Bake until the corners are bubbling, 30 to 40 minutes. Remove the foil and bake uncovered for 7 to 10 minutes, until the top is lightly browned.

7. Remove the pan from the oven, cover it with foil, and let it stand for 10 minutes. Then cut the baked penne into squares (like lasagna), and serve with extra grated cheese and warmed pasta sauce on the side, if desired.

Pizza

Make-your-own-pizza night is back, and it's fun! This dough is a great source of whole grains, and the four different flours help achieve the kind of thin and tasty crust my family loves.

SERVES 8

1 cup warm water (about 110°F), plus more if needed
2 eggs
2 tablespoons plus 2 teaspoons olive oil
1 15-ounce can chickpeas, drained and well rinsed
1¼ cups brown rice flour
1 cup sweet sorghum flour
1 cup millet flour
¾ cup potato starch
1 envelope (about 2½ teaspoons) active dry yeast
2 teaspoons salt, plus more to taste
2 teaspoons xanthan gum
Nonstick cooking spray
1 28-ounce can diced tomatoes, drained
2 cups grated part-skim mozzarella cheese
¼ cup fresh basil leaves, torn

1. Place the water, eggs, and 2 tablespoons of olive oil in a small bowl and whisk to combine. Set aside.

2. Place the chickpeas in a food processor fitted with a dough blade or in a standing mixer fitted with a dough hook, and pulse until the chickpeas are chopped, but still chunky. Add the brown rice flour, sorghum flour, millet flour, potato starch, yeast, salt, and xanthan gum. Pulse the mixture while you gradually add the

warm water mixture until the dough collects in a ball around the blade or hook.

3. Adjust the texture of the dough as necessary by adding more warm water if it's too dry, or a little flour if it's too wet, as you mix or pulse it in the processor. The dough should have a soft and supple but not sticky texture, and should spring back softly. (I like to take mine out of the processor and knead it a few times by hand to make sure the consistency is still soft but elastic.)

4. Coat a large bowl with cooking spray. Place the dough in the bowl, cover it with plastic wrap, and let it rest at room temperature until it has doubled in size, 1 to 2 hours.

5. Punch the dough down and flatten it on a pizza pan or screen. Cover the dough with a dry dish towel and let it rest for 15 to 20 minutes.

6. Meanwhile, preheat the oven to its highest temperature.

7. Remove the towel and top the dough with the tomatoes, mozzarella, and fresh basil. Sprinkle with salt to taste, and drizzle with the remaining olive oil. Bake for 15 to 20 minutes, until the crust has browned around the edges and the cheese is bubbly. Serve immediately.

Ultimate Mom tip: Double or triple this recipe and you will be ahead of the game for school parties, pizza day, or birthday bashes for your g-free kids!

Fish and Chips

When I was growing up, Friday night meals always featured fish. We often went out to a restaurant called Coffee's in Providence, Rhode Island, where the fish and chips were so good! Big fries, and great fish! No matter where you're from, I think you'll come to love my g-free version.

SERVES 4

Chips
4 large russet potatoes (about 2 pounds total)
2 tablespoons canola oil

Fish
1 5-ounce box gluten-free crackers
2 tablespoons grated Parmesan cheese
½ teaspoon gluten-free garlic powder
½ teaspoon gluten-free paprika
¼ teaspoon freshly ground black pepper
½ teaspoon salt
2 large tilapia fillets (about 1 pound total), cut in half lengthwise
2 eggs
2 tablespoons canola oil

Gluten-free ketchup, for serving (optional)

1. Preheat the oven to 350°F.

2. Prepare the chips: Peel the potatoes, cut them into ⅓-inch-thick slices, and then cut the slices into ⅓-inch-wide sticks.

3. Heat the canola oil in a large skillet over medium-high heat.

Elisabeth Hasselbeck

Working in batches, add the potatoes and fry until they begin to turn golden, about 5 minutes. Using a slotted spoon, transfer the potatoes to paper towels to drain.

4. Spread the potatoes out in a single layer in a baking pan, and bake on the top rack of the oven for about 10 minutes or until golden brown.

5. Meanwhile, prepare the fish: Place the crackers, Parmesan, garlic powder, paprika, and black pepper in a food processor, and pulse until fine crumbs form. Spread the crumbs out on a sheet of wax paper. Sprinkle the salt over the fish. Place the eggs in a shallow bowl and whisk to break up the yolks. Dip the fish pieces in the eggs and then press them in the crumbs to coat. Transfer to a plate.

6. Heat a large ovenproof skillet over medium-high heat. Add the canola oil and when it's hot, add the fish, and cook for 5 to 6 minutes, turning the pieces once, until both sides are browned. Then slide the skillet into the oven and bake for 5 to 6 minutes, until the fish flakes when pressed with a fork. Serve immediately, with the chips. Pass the ketchup if desired.

Serve the fish with my homemade tartar sauce (see page 53) to make this dish extra-special.

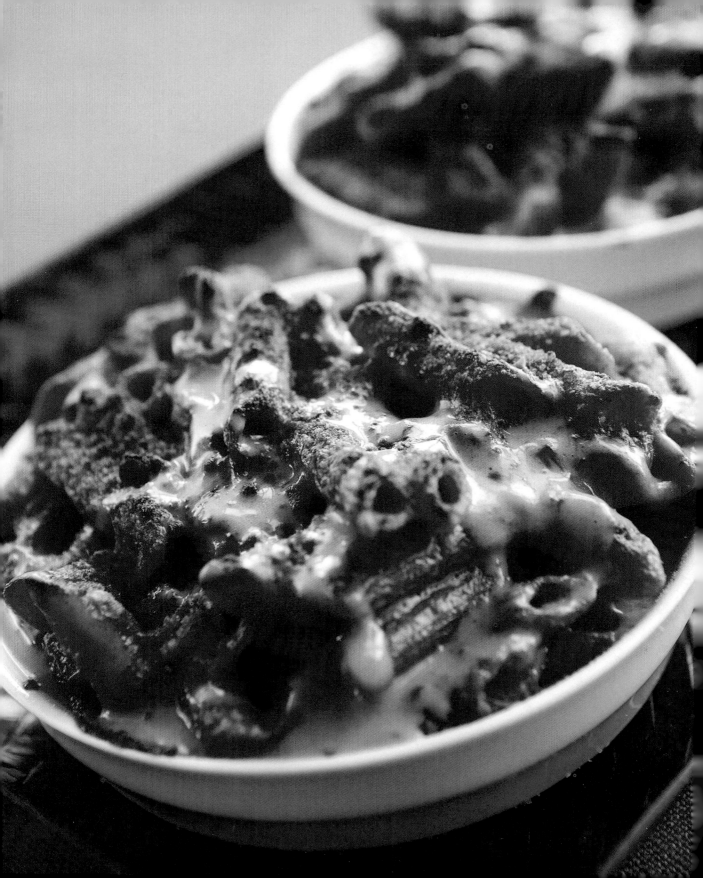

Mac and Cheese

Whoever came up with mac and cheese—the ultimate one-pot meal for picky kids—was a genius. It was a challenge to make a g-free version that could be as beloved and satisfying as the original . . . but this recipe meets the challenge and then some! Feel free to play around with the cheese/spice combo that works for your young tasters, but try it once as described below. I suspect it'll be a crowd-pleaser.

SERVES 6

1 pound gluten-free macaroni: shells, penne, or elbows
3 cups 2% milk
1 teaspoon potato starch
½ teaspoon salt
2 tablespoons salted butter
2 tablespoons gluten-free reduced-fat cream cheese
½ teaspoon gluten-free paprika
½ teaspoon gluten-free garlic powder
¼ teaspoon freshly ground black pepper (optional)
3 cups grated mild cheddar or American cheese, or a mixture

1. Bring a large pot of salted water to a boil. Add the pasta, and cook it for 3 minutes less than the package instructions indicate.

2. Meanwhile, make the sauce: Combine the milk, potato starch, and salt in a medium bowl and whisk to combine.

3. Place the butter and cream cheese in a large stockpot and heat over medium heat. When the cream cheese is soft and the butter has melted, slowly whisk in the milk mixture. Cook, stirring occasionally, until the mixture is hot and has thickened slightly, 3 to 4 minutes. Add the paprika, garlic powder, and black pepper if using. Reduce the heat to low and add the cheese. Cook, stirring frequently, until thickened, about 3 minutes.

4. Drain the pasta, add it to the sauce, and cook for 1 minute, stirring to coat the pasta with the sauce. Divide in individual serving dishes and place in a 400° oven for 10 minutes until the tops are browned. Serve, and watch them smile!

Elisabeth Hasselbeck

Seafood Chowder

This creamy, chunky chowder uses naturally gluten-free potatoes instead of flour to thicken the broth. Serve a warm hunk of cornbread alongside (see page 105) to make this a truly special meal.

SERVES 8

½ pound gluten-free bacon, finely chopped
1 yellow onion, chopped
2 celery stalks, chopped
2 garlic cloves, minced
1 tablespoon salted butter
2 pounds Yukon Gold potatoes (about 4 medium), diced
2 bay leaves
1 fresh rosemary sprig
½ teaspoon salt
½ teaspoon gluten-free paprika
¼ teaspoon freshly ground black pepper, or to taste
Pinch of ground cayenne pepper
1 pound littleneck clams, rinsed well
1 pound assorted fish, such as tuna, salmon, and tilapia, cut into 1-inch
   cubes
1 cup heavy cream
2 teaspoons gluten-free Worcestershire sauce
¼ cup chopped fresh chives

1 Place the bacon, onion, celery, garlic, and butter in a large stockpot. Cook over medium-high heat, stirring often, until the bacon browns and the celery softens, 4 to 5 minutes.

2. Add the potatoes, bay leaves, rosemary, salt, paprika, black pepper, and cayenne. Then add enough water to cover the potatoes completely, cover the pot, and bring to a steady simmer. Cook for 15 to 20 minutes, until the potatoes are fork-tender.

3. Add the clams, cover, and cook for 1 minute, until the clams open (discard any that do not open). Remove the clams, pull the meat from inside the shells, and give them a rough chop. Return the clam meat to the pot. Remove and discard the bay leaves.

4. Using a fork or a potato masher, mash about half of the potatoes in the pot. Stir the soup well to incorporate the mashed-up potato. Add the fish pieces, cover the pot, and take it off the heat. Let the soup rest for 5 minutes while the fish steams.

5. Stir in the cream and the Worcestershire sauce. Ladle the soup into bowls, sprinkle with the chives, and serve immediately.

Elisabeth Hasselbeck

Vegetable Fried Rice

This dish seems so authentic, you might have everyone at the table asking for a fortune cookie after they are finished! The ribbons of cooked egg on top add texture, protein, and color contrast.

SERVES 8

2 cups gluten-free short-grain brown rice

4 cups baby spinach

2 eggs

Nonstick cooking spray

2 tablespoons Asian sesame oil or canola oil

5 ounces shiitake mushrooms

2 carrots, thinly sliced

4 scallions, thinly sliced, using both white and green parts

1 teaspoon gluten-free red pepper flakes

2 cups fresh or frozen corn kernels

½ cup gluten-free beef broth

2 tablespoons gluten-free soy sauce

¼ cup packed fresh mint or basil leaves, torn or sliced

½ pound cooked chicken, sliced or cubed (optional)

1. Cook the rice according to the package instructions, and set it aside.

2. Heat a large skillet over high heat. Add the spinach and 1 tablespoon of water. Cook, stirring often, until the spinach wilts, about 30 seconds. Transfer the spinach to a plate.

3. Place the eggs in a small bowl and beat them with a fork. Heat a large skillet over medium-high heat, coat it with cooking spray, and add the eggs. Tilt the skillet so the eggs cover the entire inside of the pan. Cook for 30 seconds. Then flip the eggs over and cook for 30 seconds more, until the eggs are cooked through. Transfer the egg "pancake" to a cutting board and let it cool. Then slice it into thin strips and set them aside.

4. Heat the same large skillet over high heat, and add the sesame or canola oil. Add the mushrooms, carrots, spinach, scallions, and red pepper flakes. Cook, stirring occasionally, until the vegetables start to soften, 2 to 3 minutes. Add the cooked rice and the corn kernels, beef broth, and soy sauce. Cook for 1 minute more, stirring often. Fold in the mint or basil. Top with the strips of egg, and the chicken if using. Serve immediately.

Elisabeth Hasselbeck

Veggie Pad Thai

Pad Thai was always a take-out favorite of mine. I think this version is as good as you'll get in a restaurant—in fact it's fresher tasting and much lower in fat than most take-out Pad Thai (which can have as much as 34 grams of fat per serving!), so you can have a guilt-free second serving.

SERVES 4

½ pound gluten-free wide rice noodles

⅓ cup fresh lime juice

3 tablespoons gluten-free fish sauce

1 tablespoon gluten-free rice vinegar

1 tablespoon granulated sugar

1 tablespoon gluten-free sweet chili sauce

1 tablespoon canola oil

1 shallot, finely minced

2 garlic cloves, finely minced

1 teaspoon olive oil

2 eggs, lightly beaten

¼ cup unsalted roasted peanuts, coarsely chopped

2 cups bean sprouts

4 scallions, thinly sliced, using both white and green parts

½ cup packed fresh cilantro leaves, chopped

If you're a seafood fan, swap out the chicken for 1 pound of grilled or steamed shrimp.

1. Bring a large pot of salted water to a boil, and cook the noodles according to the package instructions. Drain, and set aside.

2. In a small bowl, whisk together the lime juice, ⅓ cup of

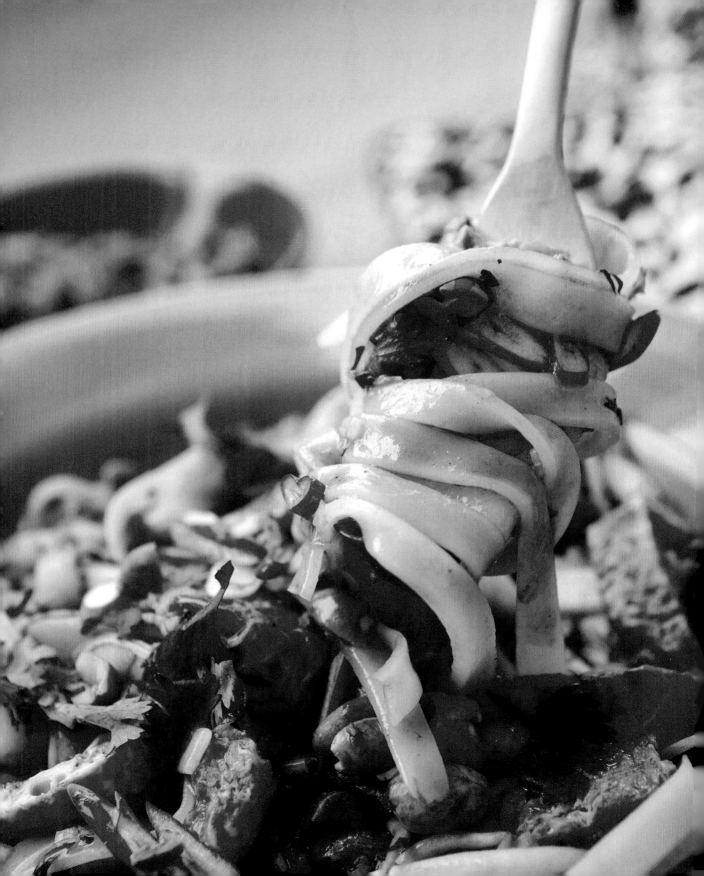

water, and the fish sauce, rice vinegar, sugar, sweet chili sauce, canola oil, shallot, and garlic. Add the warm noodles and toss.

3. Heat the olive oil in a large skillet over medium-high heat, and add the eggs. Tilt the skillet so the eggs cover the entire inside of the pan. Cook for 30 seconds. Flip the eggs over and cook for 30 seconds more, until the eggs are cooked through. Transfer the egg "pancake" to a cutting board and let it cool. Slice into thin strips and set aside. Top the noodles with the peanuts, sprouts, and scallions. Using a pair of tongs or two large spoons, toss until the noodles are evenly coated. Sprinkle with the cilantro, top with the cooked egg, and serve immediately.

{Chapter 5}

Deliciously Irresistible Desserts

With a wide variety of ingredients for the gluten-free baker now on the market, there's simply no reason to settle for bland or dry baked goods. By making my version of the classics—like Double Chocolate Brownies (page 209), Classic Yellow Cupcakes (page 194), and Chocolate Chip Cookies (page 215)—you'll quickly appreciate the wide range of great-tasting g-free flours, and happily realize that you can be reunited with all the treats you enjoyed pre-g-free. See "The Secrets of G-Free Baking" on page 15 for more tips and getting-started strategies.

Egg "Doll" Biscuits

This recipe has one of my very first memories attached to it. There I was, all of five years old, "painting" what seemed like thousands of biscuits with an egg wash and then lining them up on the counter. I quickly learned that diligent work paid off when I got to taste the first freshly baked doll biscuit of the batch. These have been made for generations in my family (my mom makes them with my daughter, Grace, every time they get together) and will be made for more to come.

MAKES 40 BISCUITS

Biscuits

Nonstick cooking spray

1 cup plus 2 tablespoons brown rice flour

⅓ cup coconut flour

⅓ cup tapioca starch

2 teaspoons baking powder

2 teaspoons guar gum

¼ cup granulated sugar

⅓ cup sweetened condensed milk

⅓ cup gluten-free solid vegetable shortening, cut into small pieces

1 egg, lightly beaten

½ teaspoon gluten-free vanilla extract

Glaze

1 cup powdered sugar

2 tablespoons 2% milk

1 teaspoon vanilla, lemon, or anise extract

Call them biscuits or call them cookies—either way, kids love helping to make them since they can roll them out with their fingers. They also make a cute holiday cookie!

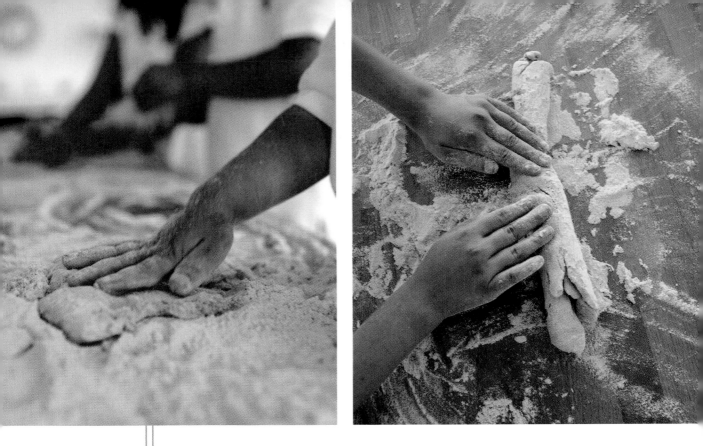

1. Bake the biscuits: Preheat the oven to 350°F. Coat three cookie sheets with nonstick spray and set them aside.

2. In a large bowl, combine 1 cup of brown rice flour and the coconut flour, tapioca starch, baking powder, guar gum, and granulated sugar. Whisk until well combined. Make a well in the center of the flour mixture and add the sweetened condensed milk, shortening, egg, and vanilla. Using a wooden spoon, stir until a thick dough forms.

3. Dust the counter with the remaining 2 tablespoons of brown rice flour. Roll the dough onto the counter and knead it with your fingers until a smooth dough forms.

4. Take a walnut-size piece of the dough, and, using your hands, roll this piece into a rope. Cross the ends of the rope to make a loop (like the breast cancer ribbon). Place the loop on one

Elisabeth Hasselbeck

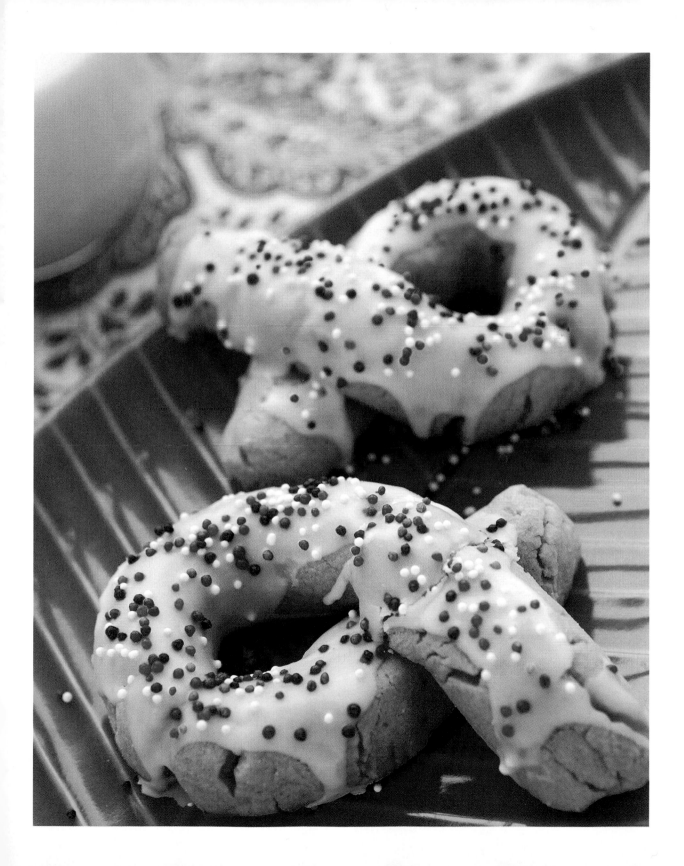

of the prepared cookie sheets, and repeat with the remaining dough, filling all three cookie sheets.

5. Place as many cookie sheets as will fit on the bottom oven rack, and bake until the biscuits are golden brown on the bottom, 3 to 5 minutes. Then move the cookie sheets to the top rack and bake until the tops are light golden brown, 3 to 5 minutes. Repeat with the remaining cookie sheets as necessary. Set the cookies aside, still on the sheets.

6. Make the glaze: Mix the powdered sugar, milk, and extract together in a small bowl until the glaze has the consistency of pancake batter.

7. While the cookies are still warm, dip the tops of the cookies in the glaze. Then set them aside on wire racks to cool completely. Store in an airtight container at room temperature for up to 5 days.

Chocolate Cashew Fudge Bars

Don't be intimidated—just because they're called "fudge" doesn't mean these dark chocolate delights are hard to make. Go gourmet with the cashews on top, or substitute your favorite topping, such as toasted coconut, white chocolate chips, or peanut butter chips.

MAKES 24 PIECES

Nonstick cooking spray
12 tablespoons (1½ sticks) salted butter, melted
1 cup finely crushed gluten-free sugar cookies (½ pound)
½ cup granulated sugar
1 5-ounce can sweetened condensed milk
1 10-ounce bag miniature marshmallows
2 10-ounce bags gluten-free semisweet chocolate chips
1 cup chopped salted cashews

1. Line a 13 × 9-inch baking pan with aluminum foil, with the ends of the foil extending over the sides. Spray the foil with cooking spray.

2. In a small bowl, mix 2 tablespoons of the melted butter with the cookie crumbs. Press this over the bottom of the prepared baking pan.

3. Place the remaining 10 tablespoons butter, the sugar, the sweetened condensed milk, and the marshmallows in a large saucepan, and cook over medium heat, stirring constantly, until the marshmallows are completely melted, 1 to 2 minutes. Then reduce the heat to low and add the chocolate chips. Cook, stirring continuously, until the chocolate is completely melted and the mixture is starting to thicken, about 1 minute. Working quickly, pour the mixture over the crumb crust, and smooth the top with a spatula.

4. Sprinkle the cashews over the top, cover with aluminum foil, and refrigerate for 2 hours or until firm. Cut into small squares. Store the fudge in an airtight container in the refrigerator for up to 2 weeks.

Elisabeth Hasselbeck

Orange Creamsicles

Hello, summer! These are so refreshing and sweet, there's no need to listen for the bell of the ice cream truck when you have some in your freezer. To make these treats dinner-party-worthy, add sections of fresh blood orange or tangerine to the orange juice layers before freezing.

MAKES 8 MINI CUPS OR POPSICLES

2 cups orange juice
2 cups gluten-free vanilla ice cream or low-fat vanilla frozen yogurt

1. Pour 2 tablespoons of the orange juice into the bottom of each of 8 small paper drinking cups or Popsicle holders. Cover, and freeze for 1 hour or until the orange juice is solid.

2. Top the frozen orange juice in each cup or Popsicle holder with ¼ cup of the vanilla ice cream or vanilla yogurt. Place in the freezer for 30 minutes to firm the ice cream or yogurt.

3. Remove from the freezer and pour the remaining orange juice over the ice cream or yogurt.

4. Freeze for at least 2 hours, or until firm, before serving. These creamsicles will keep up to six months in the freezer!

Yellow Birthday Cake or Classic Yellow Cupcakes

Birthday celebrations call for buttery cakes in my house. This cake even tastes great when made the day before; just be sure to wrap it in several layers of plastic wrap once it cools, to keep it moist. Mix and match flavors with my Trio of Icings (page 199).

MAKES 2 9-INCH ROUND CAKES OR 16 CUPCAKES

Nonstick cooking spray (for cake pans)

1 cup brown rice flour

½ cup coconut flour

½ cup tapioca starch

1 tablespoon baking powder

1 teaspoon xanthan gum

¼ teaspoon salt

1½ cups granulated sugar

1 cup 2% milk

½ cup canola or light olive oil

2 eggs, lightly beaten

2 teaspoons gluten-free vanilla extract or powder

Icing (see page 199)

If you mixed up my Power Flours (see page 17), you'll use 2 cups of the Yellow Birthday Cake baking mix (see page 23) in place of the flours listed here.

1. Preheat the oven to 350°F. Line a 12-cup muffin tin with cupcake liners or coat two 9-inch cake pans with cooking spray.

2. Place the brown rice flour, coconut flour, tapioca starch, baking powder, xanthan gum, and salt in a large bowl, and whisk to combine. Make a well in the center of the flour. Add the sugar, milk, canola or olive oil, eggs, and vanilla extract or powder. Using an electric mixer, beat on low speed for about 1 minute,

Elisabeth Hasselbeck

until the batter is very smooth. Divide the batter between the prepared cake pans, or fill each muffin cup to the top. (If making cupcakes, reserve the leftover batter and repeat with 4 more cupcake liners.)

3. *For the cake,* bake for 20 to 25 minutes, until the cakes spring back when the tops are pressed or until a toothpick tester comes out clean. *For the cupcakes,* bake for 15 to 18 minutes, until the cupcakes spring back when the tops are pressed or until a toothpick tester comes out clean. Remove the cake or cupcakes from their forms and let them cool completely on a wire rack.

4. Once the cakes or cupcakes are cool, use a small spatula or a butter knife to ice them with your favorite icing. Store in an airtight container in the refrigerator for up to 5 days.

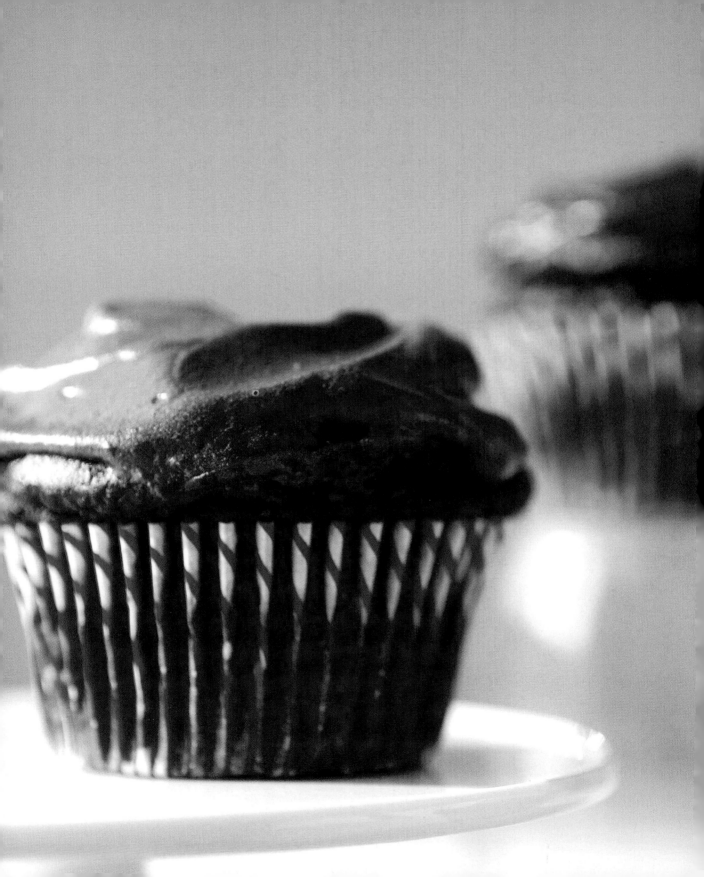

Chocolate Devil's Food Cupcakes

This dark rich cupcake will make any chocolate lover's head spin. I
live for these cupcakes! *Really, I do! Go ahead and try them yourself,
and you will see why.*

MAKES 16 CUPCAKES

1 cup boiling-hot water
1 cup gluten-free unsweetened cocoa powder
1 cup brown rice flour
½ cup sweet sorghum flour
½ cup potato flour
2 teaspoons baking soda
1 teaspoon guar gum
⅛ teaspoon salt
2 cups granulated sugar
8 tablespoons (1 stick) salted butter, at room temperature
2 eggs, at room temperature
1 teaspoon gluten-free vanilla extract
1 cup low-fat buttermilk
Icing (see page 199)

If you mixed up my Power Flours (see page 17), you'll use 2 cups of the Devil's Food baking mix (see page 23) in place of the flours listed here.

1. Preheat the oven to 400°F. Line a 12-cup muffin tin with
cupcake liners.

2. In a large bowl, whisk the hot water and cocoa powder together.

3. In another large bowl, stir together the brown rice flour,
sorghum flour, potato flour, baking soda, guar gum, and salt.

4. Add the sugar and butter to the cocoa mixture. With an
electric mixer on high speed, beat until a smooth, shiny mixture

forms, about 30 seconds. Then beat in the eggs and vanilla on low speed until incorporated.

5. Add half of the flour mixture and beat on low speed just until combined; there may be dry spots. Add ½ cup of the buttermilk, mixing on low speed until just incorporated. Repeat with the remaining flour mixture and the remaining buttermilk. Fill each muffin cup to the top with the batter. Reserve the remaining batter and fill 4 more cupcake liners; set aside. Bake for 15 to 20 minutes, until the centers of the cupcakes are firm to the touch.

6. Remove the cupcakes from the muffin tin and let them cool completely on a wire rack. Repeat with the remaining batter.

7. Once the cupcakes are cool, use a small spatula or a butter knife to ice them with your choice of icing. Store in an airtight container in the refrigerator for up to 5 days.

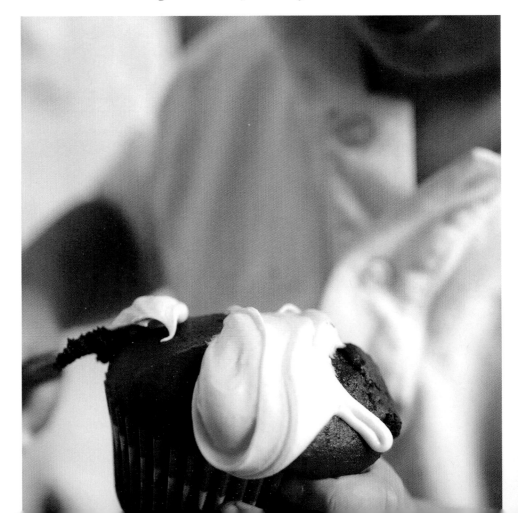

Trio of Icings

The Sophisticated Chocolate Cream Cheese

Icing *My personal favorite, this rich icing is the perfect creamy balance to the sweet cake beneath. If heaven were food, mine would be made of this icing!*

MAKES 2 CUPS

½ cup gluten-free reduced-fat cream cheese
½ cup powdered sugar
¼ cup gluten-free unsweetened cocoa powder
8 tablespoons (1 stick) salted butter, at room temperature

This icing stores well in an airtight container in the refrigerator for 3 days. Bring it to room temperature before icing your cake or cupcakes.

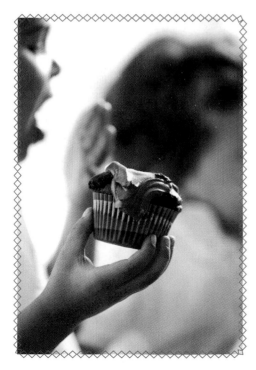

In a medium bowl, beat the cream cheese, powdered sugar, and cocoa powder together until smooth. Gradually beat in the butter until a smooth, light frosting forms. Use immediately, or cover and refrigerate for up to 3 days. Be sure to bring the icing back to room temperature before using it.

Good Times Marshmallow Filling or Icing *Devil Dogs were one of my snack-machine after-school treats when I was a kid. Full disclosure: If Devil Dogs were g-free, I would still be popping quarters into the machine at work at least once a day. This frosting will remind you of that filling and take your chocolate cake back in time!*

MAKES 2 CUPS

4 tablespoons (½ stick) unsalted butter, at room temperature
¾ cup powdered sugar
1 cup gluten-free marshmallow cream, such as Marshmallow Fluff
½ teaspoon gluten-free vanilla extract

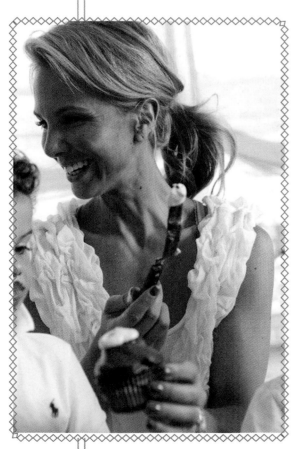

In a medium bowl, beat the butter, powdered sugar, marshmallow cream, and vanilla until smooth. Cover and refrigerate for up to 5 days. Bring the icing back to room temperature before using.

Kids' Choice Chocolate Buttercream

This is the chocolate icing choice for little ones! My chocolate-lovin' boys, Taylor and Isaiah, cannot get enough. This icing pairs well with the Yellow Birthday Cake on page 194.

MAKES 2 CUPS

8 tablespoons (1 stick) salted butter, at room temperature
½ cup gluten-free unsweetened cocoa powder
1 teaspoon gluten-free vanilla extract
1 cup powdered sugar
2 tablespoons 2% milk

1. In a large bowl, cream the butter with an electric mixer. Add the cocoa powder and vanilla. Gradually add the powdered sugar, beating well on medium speed and scraping the sides and bottom of the bowl often. When all the sugar has been mixed in, the icing will appear dry. Add the milk and beat on medium speed until the icing is light and fluffy.

2. Keep the bowl covered with a damp cloth until ready to use. For best results, also keep the bowl of icing in the refrigerator when not in use.

3. Refrigerated in an airtight container, this icing can be stored for 2 weeks. Bring back to room temperature and rewhip before using.

Banana Cream Pie

Sunny, Southern, and Soooo good! Retro desserts are always in fashion when they taste this rich and creamy. You'll make a "Top Chef" entrance when you show up at your next party with this impressive g-free dessert; they'll never forget it.

SERVES 10

Crust
1 pound gluten-free cinnamon cookies or graham crackers
4 tablespoons (½ stick) salted butter, melted

Banana Cream Filling
6 eggs, separated
3 cups 2% milk
1⅓ cups granulated sugar
2 tablespoons cornstarch
1 teaspoon gluten-free vanilla extract
¼ teaspoon salt
2 tablespoons salted butter, cut into pieces
6 ripe bananas, sliced into ¼-inch-thick rounds

Topping
½ teaspoon cream of tartar
⅓ cup superfine sugar

> *Unlike my Banana Bread (page 213), this recipe calls for bananas that are not overly ripe—you want to avoid a speckled look.*

1. Prepare the crust: Place the cookies or graham crackers in a food processor, and pulse until fine crumbs form. Drizzle the melted butter into the food processor over the cookie crumbs and

Elisabeth Hasselbeck

pulse several times to mix. Press the crumb mixture into the bottom of a 10-inch pie plate with deep sides.

2. Prepare the pie filling: Place the egg whites in a large bowl and set aside to use for the topping. Place the egg yolks in a large saucepan. Add the milk, granulated sugar, cornstarch, vanilla, and salt, and whisk well.

3. Place the saucepan over medium heat and simmer, whisking continuously, until the mixture thickens and becomes pudding-like, 2 to 3 minutes. Stir in the butter. Fold in the bananas. Pour the filling into the prepared pie plate.

4. Prepare the topping: Add the cream of tartar to the reserved egg whites, and beat with an electric mixer on high speed until soft peaks form. With the beater running, add the superfine sugar and continue beating until it is combined and the mixture is glossy, about 20 seconds. Spoon the egg whites over the filling and spread them out with a rubber spatula. Using the back of a spoon, create decorative swirls.

5. Bake the pie until the topping is golden, 10 to 15 minutes. Transfer the pie to a wire rack and let it cool completely. Then refrigerate the pie for 3 hours or more before serving.

Blueberry-Raspberry Cobbler

When it comes to dessert, I tend to reach first for the chocolate offerings. But this one has the ability to turn my head with its crisp top, cakey center, and soft fruit beneath. Delicious!

SERVES 8

Frozen berries work just as well in this recipe and are more economical than fresh. Defrost the berries in a bowl on the countertop for 30 minutes before baking.

Berries
2 pints blueberries (defrosted if frozen)
2 pints raspberries (defrosted if frozen)

Biscuit Topping
¾ cup granulated sugar
½ cup brown rice flour
¼ cup sweet sorghum flour
¼ cup coconut flour
I teaspoon baking powder
I teaspoon xanthan gum
¼ teaspoon salt
3 tablespoons cold salted butter, cut into small pieces
½ cup 2% milk

Crunchy Topping
I cup granulated sugar
2 teaspoons cornstarch
¼ teaspoon gluten-free ground cinnamon
I cup boiling water

1. Preheat the oven to 350°F.

2. Layer the blueberries and raspberries in a 9 × 13-inch baking dish.

3. Prepare the biscuit topping: Place the sugar, brown rice flour, sweet sorghum flour, coconut flour, baking powder, xanthan gum, and salt in a large bowl and stir to combine. Using your fingertips or a pastry blender, blend in the butter until the mixture resembles coarse meal. Stir in the milk until just combined. Spoon dollops of the wet dough over the blueberry-raspberry mixture. Don't smooth the dollops out.

4. Prepare the crunchy topping: In a medium bowl, combine the sugar, cornstarch, and cinnamon, and stir well. Sprinkle the cinnamon sugar over the biscuit topping. Drizzle the boiling water over the top, wetting the top of the biscuit topping and allowing the water to soak the berries.

5. Bake, uncovered, for 25 to 30 minutes, until a firm crust forms on the top and the edges are bubbly. Let the cobbler cool for 5 minutes before serving.

Chocolate Pudding

Beyond decadent. You can get creative with flavor options like peanut butter or butterscotch swirls. As for me, I simply add a spoon!

SERVES 8

4 cups whole milk

¾ cup granulated sugar

¼ cup gluten-free unsweetened cocoa powder

¼ cup cornstarch

2 teaspoons gluten-free vanilla extract

Pinch of salt

8 gluten-free vanilla or chocolate cookies, crushed

Topping the pudding with cookie crumbs keeps a skin from forming, but if you're a fan of the skin, put all the crumbs in the bottom of your dessert dish instead.

1. Combine the milk, sugar, cocoa powder, cornstarch, vanilla, and salt in a large saucepan. Place it over medium-low heat and cook, whisking often, until the mixture thickens, 3 to 4 minutes. If lumps start to form, reduce the heat to low and whisk well to break up the lumps.

2. Set out 8 ramekins or dessert dishes, and sprinkle half of the cookie crumbs into them. Spoon ½ cup of the pudding over the crumbs in each dish, and top with the remaining crumbs.

3. Cover and refrigerate for at least 3 hours before serving. (The pudding will keep in the refrigerator for up to 3 days.)

Chocolate Pudding Pops

Chocolate pudding pops are my absolute favorite summertime treat. Confession: I hide two in the way back of the freezer so I can enjoy their decadence by myself as soon as the kids are in bed.

MAKES 2½ CUPS, OR 10 POPSICLES

6 large egg yolks

⅔ cup granulated sugar

½ cup gluten-free unsweetened cocoa powder

¼ cup cornstarch

2 teaspoons gluten-free vanilla extract

¼ teaspoon salt

2 cups whole milk

Reserve the unused egg whites from this recipe, refrigerate them in an airtight container, and use them for another recipe, such as the Angel Food Cake on page 226. Egg whites will keep for up to 1 week in the fridge.

1. Place the egg yolks, sugar, cocoa powder, cornstarch, vanilla, and salt in a medium heatproof bowl, and whisk until a thick, smooth paste forms. Set aside.

2. Bring the milk to a slow boil in a medium saucepan over medium heat. Remove from the heat and quickly whisk ¼ cup of the hot milk into the egg mixture (so the eggs don't curdle). Repeat. Then add all the remaining milk to the egg mixture and whisk well. Return the mixture to the saucepan and cook over very low heat, whisking continuously until the mixture thickens to a heavy cream consistency, about 1 minute.

3. Remove from the heat and whisk to break up any soft curds that might have formed from the cornstarch. The mixture will resemble a thick icing. Divide it among ten ¼-cup Popsicle molds or small paper drinking cups. Cover, and freeze for at least 3 hours or until firm before serving. These pudding pops will keep for up to 6 months in the freezer.

Chocolate Almond Bark

This makes a great gift: just bake, box, and bring! If you're not an almond fan, substitute dried cherries, raisins, or marshmallows—any add-in as long as it's g-free!

SERVES 10

1 pound gluten-free semisweet chocolate
2 cups whole almonds, toasted and coarsely chopped

1. Line a 13 × 9-baking dish with parchment paper.

2. Grate enough of the chocolate to make 2 tablespoons, and then chop the rest.

3. Heat the chopped chocolate in the top of a double boiler set over simmering water, stirring frequently, until almost melted. Remove the top pan from the heat and stir the chocolate continuously for about 1 minute. Then let the chocolate cool completely in the pan, stirring occasionally, about 30 minutes.

4. Add the grated chocolate to the cooled melted chocolate. Return the top pan to the simmering water and stir constantly over medium-low heat until the temperature of the chocolate reaches 90°F or until most of the grated chocolate has melted completely. Then remove the top pan and stir in the almonds.

5. Dry the outside of the top pan so no water will drip from it into the chocolate. Pour the chocolate mixture into the prepared baking dish and smooth the top with a rubber spatula. Cool on the countertop, uncovered, for 30 minutes. Then cover with aluminum foil and refrigerate until hardened, about 45 minutes.

6. Using a sharp knife, slice the chocolate block into uneven pieces for bark. Serve immediately, or store the bark in an airtight container in the refrigerator for up to 2 weeks.

Elisabeth Hasselbeck

Double Chocolate Brownies

So *worth waiting for! I am confident that these are the best brownies you will ever taste. The black bean flour is the secret-agent ingredient that keeps the brownies moist instead of crumbly. My mom, a.k.a. "the brownie maker in chief," approves!*

If you want to make a double batch of these, invest in two 8 × 8-inch baking pans. The brownies don't always bake well in the center if you double the batch and bake it in a 13 × 9-inch pan.

MAKES 12 BROWNIES

Nonstick cooking spray

6 tablespoons salted butter, cut into 4 pieces

4 ounces gluten-free bittersweet chocolate, finely chopped, or ¾ cup gluten-free bittersweet chocolate chips

1 cup granulated sugar

¼ teaspoon salt

⅓ cup unsweetened applesauce

2 large eggs, at room temperature, lightly beaten

1 teaspoon gluten-free vanilla extract

¾ cup sweet white rice flour

¼ cup potato starch

¼ cup black bean flour

¼ cup gluten-free unsweetened cocoa powder

1 teaspoon baking powder

1 teaspoon xanthan gum

1 cup gluten-free milk chocolate chunks

If you mixed up my Power Flours (see page 17), you'll use 1¼ cups of the Brownies baking mix in place of the rice flour, potato starch, and black bean flour listed here.

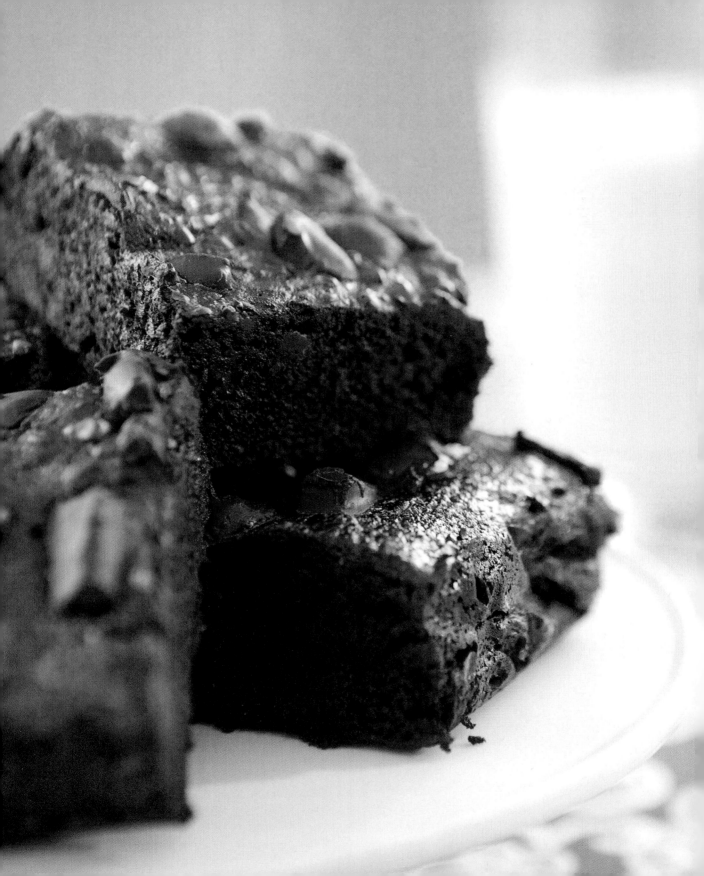

1. Preheat the oven to 325°F. Coat an 8-inch square baking dish with nonstick spray.

2. In a medium saucepan set over low heat, combine the butter and bittersweet chocolate. Warm, stirring often, until melted, about 2 minutes. Remove from the heat and stir in the sugar and salt. Add the applesauce, eggs, and vanilla, and stir until well blended. Sprinkle the white rice flour, potato starch, black bean flour, cocoa powder, baking powder, and xanthan gum over the mixture and stir until just blended. Stir in the chocolate chunks.

3. Pour the batter into the prepared baking dish and spread it out evenly. Bake until a toothpick inserted into the center of the brownies comes out almost completely clean, 25 to 30 minutes.

4. Transfer the pan to a wire rack and let the brownies cool completely. Then cut into 2-inch squares and serve.

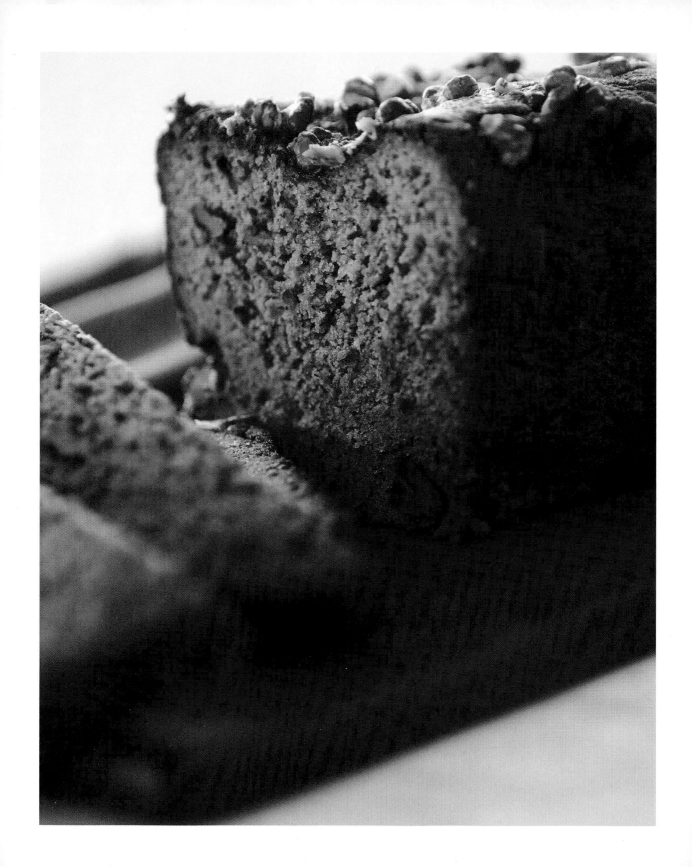

Banana Bread

My mom's banana bread always made the house smell so good! No one will suspect that this one is g-free; I love it as much as ever. Keep in mind that the ripest bananas make the moistest bread.

SERVES 10

Nonstick cooking spray
5 tablespoons unsalted butter, at room temperature
1 cup granulated sugar
2 eggs
1½ cups mashed banana (about 4 small very ripe bananas)
1 cup brown rice flour
¾ cup millet flour
1 teaspoon baking soda
½ teaspoon salt
½ teaspoon xanthan gum
¼ teaspoon baking powder
½ cup chopped walnuts (optional)

1. Preheat the oven to 350°F. Line a 2-pound loaf pan with aluminum foil and then coat the foil with cooking spray.

2. Place the butter and sugar in a large bowl. With an electric mixer on high speed, beat until the mixture is light yellow and fluffy. Add the eggs, one at a time, mixing on medium speed until combined.

3. Add the mashed banana and ⅓ cup of water, and mix on low speed for 1 minute. Sprinkle the brown rice flour, millet flour, baking soda, salt, xanthan gum, and baking powder over the bananas. If you are adding nuts, add them to the bowl and then, using a wooden spoon, stir the mixture until just combined.

4. Spoon the batter into the prepared loaf pan, and bake until the center of the bread springs back to the touch, 50 to 55 minutes. (If the bread starts to brown too quickly on the top, cover it loosely with a piece of aluminum foil.)

5. Transfer the loaf pan to a wire rack and let it cool for 5 minutes. Then lift the bread out of the pan and let it cool completely on the wire rack before slicing. Wrapped tightly in aluminum foil, the bread will keep for up to 5 days in the refrigerator.

Elisabeth Hasselbeck

Chocolate Chip Cookies

The chocolate chip cookie—what could be more American? After what seemed like hundreds of tests, I've found the ideal g-free version: perfectly chewy, not too crumbly, loaded with chips, and deliciously tasty. You will fool them with this, trust me! Serve now, disclose later.

MAKES 4 DOZEN COOKIES

Nonstick cooking spray
1½ cups brown rice flour
½ cup potato flour
¼ cup tapioca starch
¼ cup millet flour
1 teaspoon baking soda
1 teaspoon xanthan gum
½ teaspoon baking powder
¼ teaspoon salt
1 cup (2 sticks) salted butter, at room temperature
1 cup packed gluten-free light brown sugar
¾ cup granulated sugar
2 eggs, lightly beaten
1 teaspoon gluten-free vanilla extract
1 12-ounce package gluten-free bittersweet chocolate chunks

If you mixed up my Power Flours (see page 17), you'll use 2½ cups of the Chocolate Chip Cookies baking mix in place of the flours listed here.

1. Preheat the oven to 350°F. Coat three cookie sheets with nonstick spray.

2. Place the brown rice flour, potato flour, tapioca starch, millet flour, baking soda, xanthan gum, baking powder, and salt in a medium-size bowl. Stir until well combined, and set aside.

3. Place the butter, brown sugar, and granulated sugar in a large bowl. Using an electric mixer, beat on medium speed until the mixture is light brown and fluffy. Add the eggs and vanilla, and beat again on medium speed until just combined.

4. Sprinkle the flour mixture over the butter mixture, and add the chocolate chunks. Using a wooden spoon, stir until a soft dough forms, about 10 turns of the spoon. Using a tablespoon measure, drop the dough onto the prepared cookie sheets, spacing them 2 inches apart.

5. Bake for 8 to 10 minutes, until the edges are lightly browned but the centers are still soft. Cool for 2 minutes on the cookie sheets before transferring the cookies to a wire rack to cool completely. Store in an airtight container at room temperature for up to 5 days, or transfer to a zipper-lock bag and freeze for up to 6 months.

Mini "Hello Mellow" Dogs

Did I mention that I loved Devil Dogs back in the day? When I went g-free, I sometimes missed that favorite childhood treat. But now you can join me in devouring the g-free version, which is just as moist and delicious—minus the cellophane packaging.

MAKES 24 INDIVIDUAL CAKES

Nonstick cooking spray

Filling
8 tablespoons (1 stick) salted butter
1 cup gluten-free marshmallow cream, such as Marshmallow Fluff
½ cup powdered sugar
½ teaspoon gluten-free vanilla extract

Cake
¾ cup brown rice flour
2 tablespoons potato starch
6 tablespoons gluten-free unsweetened cocoa powder
½ teaspoon baking soda
½ teaspoon xanthan gum
3 tablespoons salted butter
1 cup granulated sugar
1 egg white
½ cup 2% milk

1. Preheat the oven to 400°F. Coat three baking sheets with nonstick spray.
2. Place the butter, marshmallow cream, and powdered sugar

in a small bowl, and beat with an electric mixer on high speed until smooth. Add the vanilla, and beat until well combined. Set the filling aside.

3. Place the brown rice flour, potato starch, cocoa powder, baking soda, and xanthan gum in a large bowl and whisk to combine.

4. Place the butter and granulated sugar in a large bowl and beat with an electric mixer on high speed until well combined. Add the egg white and beat until a thick, light-colored mixture forms. Add half of the flour mixture and beat until just combined. Add ¼ cup of the milk and beat on low speed. Repeat, adding the remaining flour and milk. Scoop the batter into a large zipper-lock bag, and press the batter into one corner of the bag. Clip ¼ inch off a corner of the bag to make a piping bag.

5. Squeeze out 4-inch lines of the batter, spaced 1 inch apart, on the prepared baking sheets (16 per sheet). Bake until the centers spring back to the touch, 5 to 7 minutes. Transfer the cakes to a wire rack and let them cool completely.

6. Spread the marshmallow cream filling over half of the cakes, and top with the remaining cakes. Serve immediately or store in an airtight container in the refrigerator for up to 3 days.

Creamy Cheesecake with Berry Topping

The first time I served this to Tim and the kids, I knew I'd hit a home run when I looked across the table and saw Grace (our food critic, with a most sophisticated palate) with her eyes closed, head waving back and forth, smiling and murmuring "Mmmmmmmm." That said it all.

Top this luscious cheesecake with the Cherry Topping or with fresh berries.

SERVES 10

Nonstick cooking spray

½ pound gluten-free cinnamon graham crackers

3 tablespoons salted butter, melted

4 8-ounce packages reduced-fat cream cheese, at room temperature

1 cup granulated sugar

1 teaspoon gluten-free vanilla extract

1 teaspoon grated lemon zest

2 eggs

2 egg whites

Cherry Topping (recipe follows)

To avoid those pesky lumps that sometimes appear in cheesecake batter, be sure that you set the cream cheese out on the counter at least 1 hour before baking so it is at room temperature.

1. Preheat the oven to 325°F. Coat a 9-inch springform pan with nonstick spray, and set it aside.

2. Break the graham crackers into small pieces and place them in a food processor or mini-chopper. Pulse 5 to 6 times, or until the crackers break apart into fine crumbs. Pour the crumbs into a bowl, and stir in the melted butter.

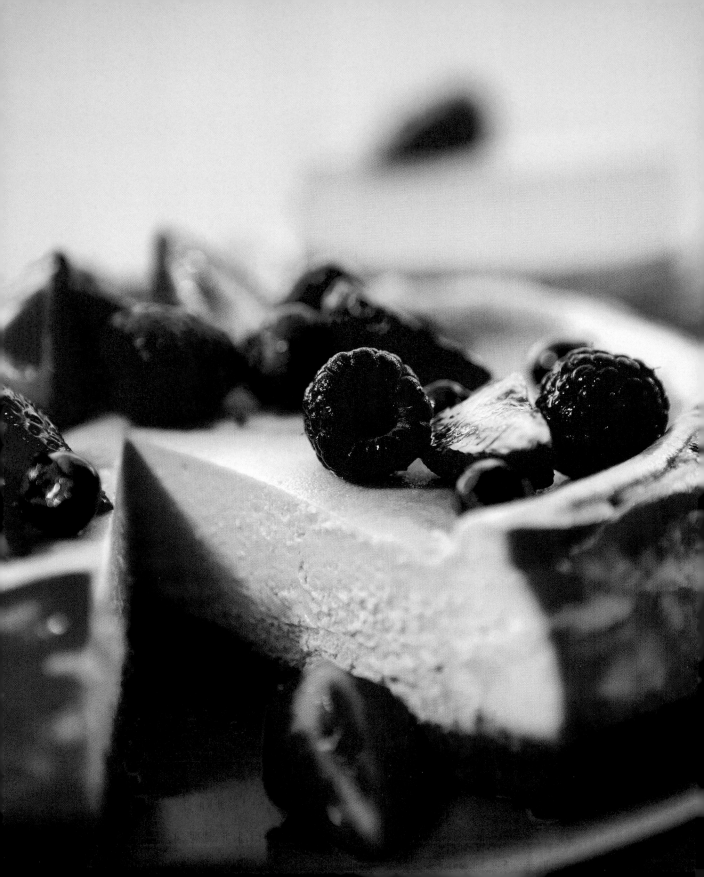

3. Press the graham cracker mixture into the bottom of the prepared springform pan.

4. Using a standing mixer or handheld mixer, beat the cream cheese in a large bowl until smooth. Add the sugar, vanilla, and lemon zest, and mix until well blended. Add the eggs and egg whites, one at a time, mixing on low speed after each addition just until blended. Pour the mixture over the crust in the springform pan, and smooth the top with a spatula. Bake for 40 to 50 minutes, until the center is almost set. Cover and refrigerate for 4 hours before serving.

5. When you are ready to serve, remove the sides of the spring-form pan, and spoon berries or the cherry topping over the cheesecake.

Cherry Topping

1 10-ounce bag frozen black cherries
Juice of 1 lemon (about 2 tablespoons)
2 teaspoons cornstarch

1. Place the cherries, lemon juice, and cornstarch in a small saucepan. Add ½ cup of water, and stir well. Bring to a boil. Immediately reduce the heat to a simmer and cook, stirring occasionally, until the mixture thickens, 5 to 6 minutes.

2. Remove the pan from the heat and let the topping cool to room temperature. Then transfer it to an airtight container and refrigerate until cold, at least 1 hour.

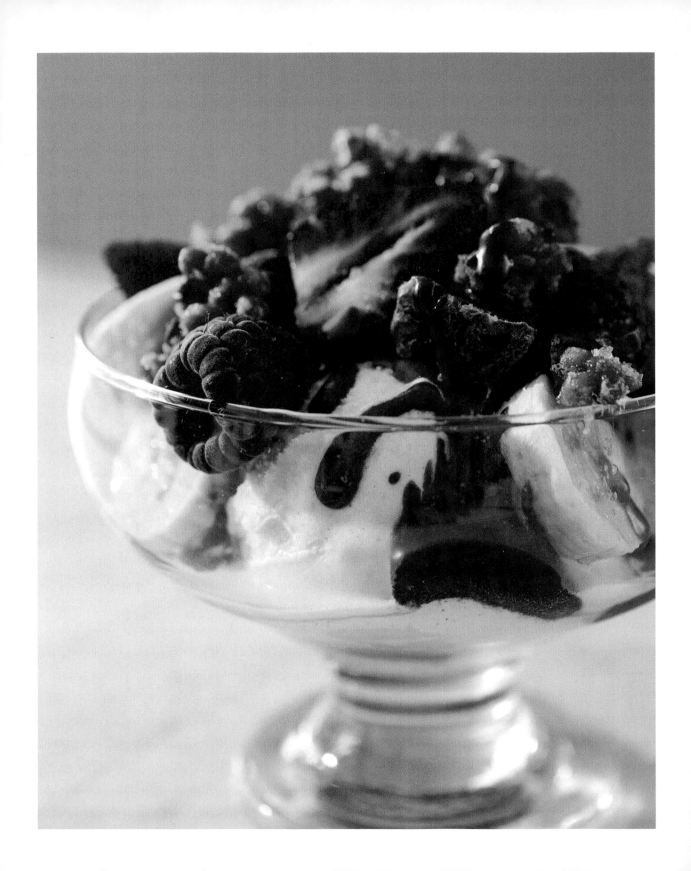

NoGii Crumble Hot Fudge Sundaes

When I was developing the recipe for my NoGii High Protein and NoGii Super Protein bars, I had the great taste of ice cream toppers in mind. Turns out the bars are the perfect g-free match for desserts as well, with crunch, chocolate, and nuts.

SERVES 4

½ cup gluten-free bittersweet chocolate chips
½ cup half-and-half
6 tablespoons powdered sugar
2 cups gluten-free vanilla frozen yogurt
2 cups sliced strawberries, bananas, or raspberries
2 NoGii High Protein bars, finely chopped

1. Make the hot fudge sauce: Place the chocolate chips and half-and-half in a small saucepan, and cook over low heat, stirring often, until the chocolate has melted, 1 to 2 minutes Whisk in the powdered sugar and set aside.

2. Assemble the sundaes: Set out four parfait glasses, and fill each one with ½ cup of the vanilla frozen yogurt. Top with the strawberries, bananas, or raspberries. Sprinkle the chopped NoGii bars over the fruit, and spoon the chocolate sauce over the top. Serve immediately.

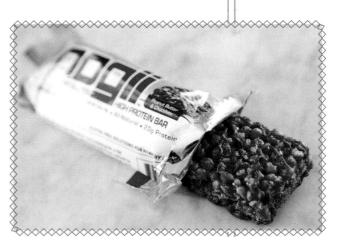

Tiramisu

You'll say "Tutti bene" when you taste this version of tiramisu. Classic tiramisu is made with raw egg yolks and whites, but in this recipe there are no comparable food-handling worries.

SERVES 10

1 pint heavy cream, chilled
2 teaspoons gluten-free vanilla extract
1 cup superfine sugar
2 pounds mascarpone cheese, at room temperature
1 cup powdered sugar
¼ cup instant espresso granules
¼ cup dark rum (optional)
10 ounces gluten-free ladyfingers
¼ cup gluten-free unsweetened cocoa powder
2 ounces gluten-free bittersweet chocolate

Freeze this for a cool dessert that's ideal for a summer dinner party. Just cover the assembled tiramisu in the baking dish with several layers of aluminum foil. Freeze until firm, about 2 hours. The tiramisu can be stored this way in the freezer for up to 3 months.

1. Chill the bowl of a standing mixer, or a large metal mixing bowl, in the freezer for 10 minutes.

2. Pour the heavy cream and the vanilla into the chilled bowl, and beat in the standing mixer or with a handheld mixer on high speed for 3 to 4 minutes, or until the cream triples in volume and is light and fluffy. With the mixer's motor running, pour in the superfine sugar and beat until just incorporated. Carefully fold in one fourth of the marscapone, using a rubber spatula. Repeat until all the mascarpone is incorporated. Refrigerate the filling while you make the base.

3. Place the powdered sugar, instant espresso, 1 cup warm water, and the rum, if using, in a large shallow bowl; stir well. Place half of the ladyfingers in the bowl and let them soak, turn-

Elisabeth Hasselbeck

ing them once, for about 10 seconds per side. Transfer them to a 13 × 9-inch baking dish. Spoon half of the mascarpone mixture over the ladyfingers. Soak the remaining ladyfingers for 10 seconds per side, and layer them over the mascarpone. Spoon the remaining mascarpone over the top and smooth with a spatula. Cover with plastic wrap or aluminum foil, and refrigerate for at least 6 hours or up to overnight.

4. When you are ready to serve the tiramisu, run a small knife around the inside edge of the baking dish to loosen the sides. Using a fine-mesh sieve, dust the top with the cocoa powder. Working over a sheet of wax paper, run a potato peeler along the squares of chocolate to make shavings. Sprinkle the chocolate shavings over the cocoa powder. Cut the tiramisu into portions, and serve directly from the baking dish.

Angel Food Cake with Mini Chocolate Chips

Tim and the kids love angel food cake, so I used to make it just for them. Even so, the glutenous baking mixes were a bit of a hazard for me—the fine powdery texture somehow often ended up getting into my nose or mouth during the mixing process. Now I make this version that we all can share, and it makes its way safely and deliciously into my mouth. I sometimes call it "Dalmatian Dog Bread" because the chocolate chips look like the dog's spots! Serve it on a red plate, pass around fireman's hats for all, turn on Disney's classic 101 Dalmatians, *and you have a party!*

SERVES 10

1¼ cups superfine sugar
½ cup sweet white rice flour
¼ cup coconut flour
¼ cup tapioca starch
1 teaspoon xanthan gum
¼ teaspoon salt
1 cup gluten-free bittersweet mini chocolate chips
14 egg whites, at room temperature
1 tablespoon gluten-free vanilla extract
1½ teaspoons cream of tartar

Superfine sugar is similar to granulated white sugar—only a smaller crystal. Most national supermarkets carry it.

1. Preheat the oven to 350°F. Line the base of a 10-inch angel food cake pan with parchment paper.

Elisabeth Hasselbeck

2. Place 1 cup of the superfine sugar in a large bowl. Add the white rice flour, coconut flour, tapioca starch, xanthan gum, and salt. Whisk until well combined. Stir in the chocolate chips and set aside.

3. In another large bowl, beat the egg whites with an electric mixer on high speed until they are frothy, about 5 seconds. Add the vanilla and cream of tartar and beat on high speed for 3 to 4 minutes, until soft peaks form. With the mixer running, gradually pour in the remaining ¼ cup superfine sugar and beat until soft, glossy peaks form.

4. Add one fourth of the flour mixture to the egg whites. With a rubber spatula, fold the flour into the whites, lifting the whites gently from the bottom of the bowl so you don't crush them. Repeat in three more additions, until all the flour is combined.

5. Spoon the batter into the prepared angel food cake pan, and bake for 45 to 50 minutes, until the top of the cake springs back to the touch. Let the cake cool for 5 minutes in the pan; then run a knife between the cake and the pan, including the tube in the center. Turn the cake out onto a wire rack and let it cool completely.

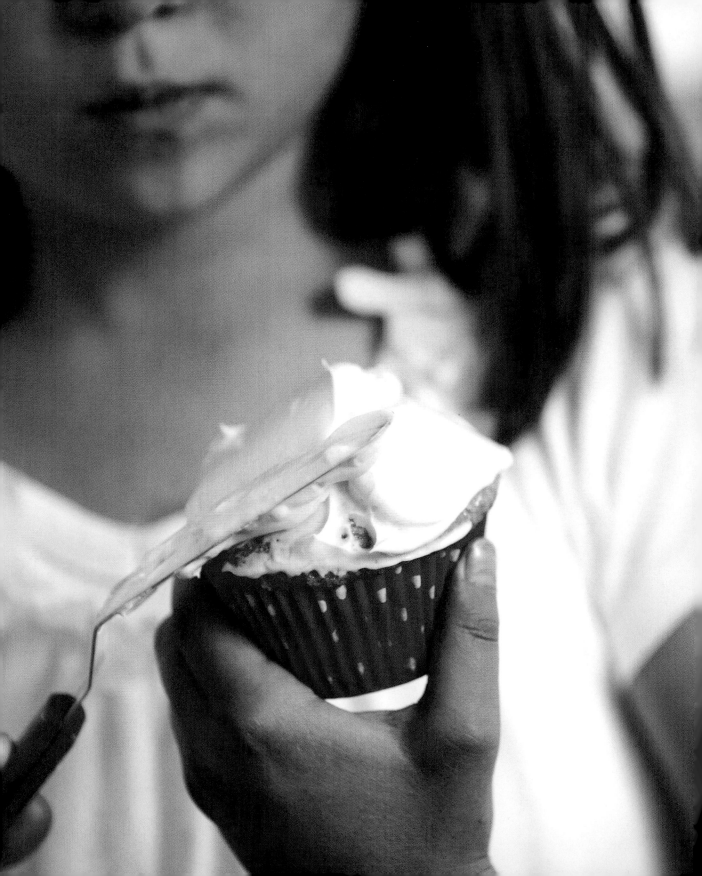

Orange Cream Cupcakes

You will love this combination of tart orange and sweet cake—every bite is a little surprise. You can also make mini-cupcakes with this batter; just bake them for 3 to 4 fewer minutes.

MAKES 12 CUPCAKES

Cupcakes

1 cup brown rice flour

½ cup coconut flour

⅓ cup tapioca starch

2 teaspoons baking powder

¼ teaspoon xanthan gum

¼ teaspoon salt

1 cup granulated sugar

½ cup canola oil

2 eggs

Grated zest and juice of 1 orange

½ teaspoon gluten-free orange extract

½ cup 2% milk

Icing

1 8-ounce package gluten-free reduced-fat cream cheese, at room temperature

½ cup powdered sugar

½ cup gluten-free light sour cream

Using citrus in baked goods can make them incredibly moist— a boon for the g-free baker!

1. Make the cupcakes: Preheat the oven to 350°F. Line a 12-cup muffin tin with cupcake liners.

2. In a medium bowl, combine the brown rice flour, coconut flour, tapioca starch, baking powder, xanthan gum, and salt. Whisk until well combined, and set aside.

3. In a large bowl, beat the sugar and canola oil together with an electric mixer on medium speed. Beat in the eggs, one at a time, until a thick, smooth yellow mixture forms.

4. Combine the orange zest, orange juice, and orange extract with the milk in a small bowl. Add half of the milk mixture to the egg mixture, and beat on low speed until just combined. Add half of the flour mixture and beat just until combined. Repeat with the remaining milk and flour mixtures. Divide the batter evenly among the prepared muffin cups.

5. Bake for 15 to 20 minutes, until the cupcakes spring back when the tops are pressed or until a toothpick tester comes out clean. Remove the cupcakes from the muffin tin and let them cool completely on a wire rack.

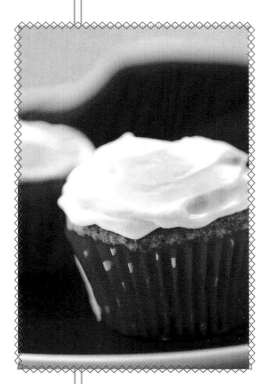

6. Make the icing: In a medium bowl, beat the cream cheese and powdered sugar together until smooth. Gradually beat in the sour cream.

7. Once the cupcakes are cool, use a small spatula or butter knife to spread the icing over the tops. Store the cupcakes in an airtight container in the refrigerator for up to 5 days.

Elisabeth Hasselbeck

Buckeyes

Both Tim and I have roots in the Buckeye State: my dad's family hails from Cleveland, and Tim's family all come from Cincinnati. This recipe is therefore a dual-family favorite. My mother-in-law, Betsy, taught me how to make buckeyes, and we serve them up during football season and most holidays.

MAKES 4 DOZEN BUCKEYES

4 tablespoons (½ stick) salted butter, at room temperature
1 cup gluten-free creamy peanut butter or soy nut butter
2 teaspoons gluten-free ground cinnamon (optional)
½ teaspoon gluten-free vanilla extract
2 cups powdered sugar
16 ounces gluten-free bittersweet chocolate, chopped (about 1 cup)

These are best straight out of the refrigerator: make them and freeze them!

1. Cover two plates with a layer of wax paper, and set aside.

2. Place the butter in a large bowl, and mash it until smooth. Add the peanut or soy nut butter, cinnamon, if using, and vanilla. Stir to combine. Transfer the mixture to a large bowl and stir in the powdered sugar; a crumbly dough will form. Roll the dough into 48 1-inch balls.

3. Melt the chopped chocolate in the top of a double boiler or in a heatproof bowl set over a pan of barely simmering water, stirring frequently until it is smooth and just warm to the touch, about 1 minute. Turn off the heat under the water.

4. Dip the peanut butter or soy nut balls into the melted chocolate, leaving a small portion of peanut butter showing at the top, and immediately transfer them to the prepared plates. Refrigerate until ready to serve.

5. To freeze, transfer the buckeyes to an air-tight container and freeze at least 2 hours, or until firm. Store in the freezer for up to 6 months.

Elisabeth Hasselbeck

Chapter 6

Get Fit with G-Free

I have never liked the expression "You are what you eat." But if it were true, I'd rather be made of cookies than of asparagus! As a child with a very active lifestyle, I didn't think much about the relative health benefits of different foods, and my parents didn't have to emphasize it either—we just ate real and home-cooked food.

That said, we all now know that the combination of eating well and exercising is the key to good and lasting health. So I try to work out regularly, and I fuel my body with many of the dishes in this book and from this chapter in particular. These calorie-friendly, get-fit meals are the perfect way to recharge your body with serious nutrients, give your skin a healthy glow, and have you feeling fantastic!

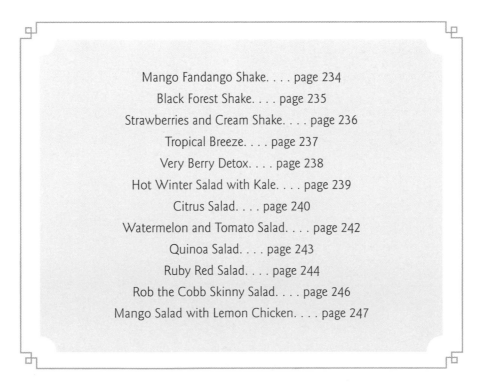

Mango Fandango Shake

My younger son, Isaiah, loves this shake because it's candy-sweet. It's a hit with me because it's a snack or a breakfast that I can make in minutes and provides 200 percent of my needs for vitamins A and C, with a hit of potassium and calcium to boot.

SERVES 1

1 large ripe mango, peeled, pitted, and cubed
½ cup plain nonfat Greek yogurt
¼ cup orange juice
¼ cup carrot juice
4 ice cubes

Place all the ingredients in a blender and blend on high speed until smooth. Serve immediately.

Nutrition stats (2 cups): 263 calories, 13 g protein, 53 g carbohydrates, 1 g fat (0 g saturated), 37 mg cholesterol, 4 g fiber, 62 mg sodium.

Elisabeth Hasselbeck

Black Forest Shake

Chocolate, cherries . . . chug! HAPPY *in a cup! I named this shake "Black Forest" because it combines chocolate and cherries, just like the classic chocolate cherry cake that hails from the Black Forest region of Germany.*

SERVES 1

1 cup frozen cherries
1½ cups skim milk
½ ripe Hass avocado, pitted and peeled
2 tablespoons gluten-free unsweetened cocoa powder
2 tablespoons gluten-free light brown sugar
4 ice cubes

No one would guess that this sweet breakfast treat also has a whopping 11 grams of fiber. That's 60 percent of your needs for the day!

Place all the ingredients in a blender and blend on high speed until smooth. Serve immediately.

Nutrition stats (2 cups): 434 calories, 17 g protein, 69 g carbohydrates, 12 g fat (2 g saturated), 7 mg cholesterol, 11 g fiber, 207 mg sodium.

Strawberries and Cream Shake

This shake tastes like a lighter version of a fast-food shake, only it's packed with protein—nearly half your needs for the day—and is very low in fat.

SERVES 1

1½ cups fresh or frozen strawberries
1 8-ounce container plain 2% yogurt
¼ cup skim milk or gluten-free vanilla soy milk
2 tablespoons granulated sugar
1 teaspoon gluten-free vanilla extract
4 ice cubes

Place all the ingredients in a blender and blend on high speed until smooth. Serve immediately.

Nutrition stats (3 cups): 368 calories, 23 g protein, 57 g carbohydrates, 5 g fat (3 g saturated), 15 mg cholesterol, 4 g fiber, 90 mg sodium.

Elisabeth Hasselbeck

Tropical Breeze

Potassium is essential for healthy muscles and proper hydration. This shake gives you half of your daily needs, making it the ideal after-workout drink.

SERVES 1

1 cup coconut water
2 bananas, peeled
1 cup cubed pineapple
Grated zest and juice of 1 lime
2 tablespoons flax meal
4 ice cubes

Place all the ingredients in a blender and blend on high speed until smooth. Serve immediately.

Nutrition stats (2 cups): 415 calories, 7 g protein, 89 g carbohydrates, 7 g fat (1 g saturated), 0 mg cholesterol, 14 fiber, 260 mg sodium.

Very Berry Detox

This sweet drink is fabulously full of fiber (19 grams), which will help you feel full even though you'll be slimming down. The spinach gives you a nutrition boost of iron, vitamin A, and folate.

SERVES 1

½ cup blueberries
½ cup raspberries
½ cup blackberries
½ cup baby spinach leaves
1 cup brewed red bush or green tea
1 tablespoon granulated sugar
4 ice cubes

   Place all the ingredients in a blender and blend on high speed until smooth. Serve immediately.

Nutrition stats (3 cups): 263 calories, 5 g protein, 63 g carbohydrates, 12 g fat (0 g saturated), 0 mg cholesterol, 19 g fiber, 25 mg sodium.

Elisabeth Hasselbeck

Hot Winter Salad with Kale

There's nothing like a crisp, fresh salad in the summertime . . . and a

warm, hearty one in the winter. I make this dish with my daughter,

Grace. She loves the way the salt brings out the sweet flavor in the red

pepper.

SERVES 4

2 tablespoons olive oil

I pound kale, chopped

2 red bell peppers, seeded and thinly sliced

¼ teaspoon salt

¼ teaspoon freshly ground black pepper

I 15-ounce can reduced-sodium red kidney beans, drained and well rinsed

I ripe Hass avocado, pitted and peeled, or I cup pureed cooked acorn
  squash

1. Heat a large skillet over high heat, and add the olive oil. Add the kale, bell peppers, salt, and black pepper, and cook until the kale is soft, 4 to 5 minutes.

2. Add the red kidney beans and the avocado or squash. Stir, and serve immediately.

Nutrition stats (2 cups): 413 calories, 18 g protein, 58 g carbohydrates, 14 g fat (2 g saturated), 0 mg cholesterol, 18 g fiber, 639 mg sodium.

Citrus Salad

Vitamin-rich greens and citrus are the basis for this sweet-tart salad. Add grilled sliced chicken to turn this healthful salad into the perfect ladies' lunch or Mother's Day brunch, and you'll add a dose of protein as well.

SERVES 4

1 bunch broccolini (about 1 pound)
½ pound mesclun salad greens
2 oranges, peeled, seeded, and sectioned
1 large pink grapefruit, peeled, seeded, and sectioned
1 Hass avocado, pitted, peeled, and cubed
½ cup slivered almonds, toasted
2 tablespoons gluten-free light mayonnaise
1 tablespoon honey
Juice of 1 orange
2 garlic cloves, minced
½ teaspoon salt

1. Pour 1 inch of water into a small saucepan, and bring it to a boil. Add the broccolini and simmer for 2 to 3 minutes, until the stems are fork-tender. Drain, and rinse the broccolini under cold running water.

2. Toss the mesclun, orange sections, grapefruit, avocado, almonds, and the broccolini in a large bowl. Set aside.

Elisabeth Hasselbeck

3. Place the mayonnaise, honey, orange juice, garlic, and salt in a blender or mini processor, and process until smooth. Drizzle the dressing over the salad, and serve immediately.

Nutrition stats (2 cups): 295 calories, 8 g protein, 40 g carbohydrates, 14 g fat (1 g saturated), 2 mg cholesterol, 10 g fiber, 394 mg sodium.

Watermelon and Tomato Salad

Re-fresh and Re-energize with the reds! Two red lycopene-rich foods create this sweet-and-salt combo that is very calorie-friendly.

SERVES 4

This is the perfect cool summertime salad. Add cooked shrimp to make it protein-rich.

4 cups mesclun greens

4 large tomatoes, sliced

4 cups sliced or chopped watermelon

Juice of 2 limes

½ teaspoon salt

¼ pound feta cheese, crumbled

¼ cup salted macadamia nuts, chopped

1. Place the mesclun greens, tomatoes, watermelon, lime juice, and salt in a large salad bowl. Toss gently to combine.

2. Sprinkle the feta and the macadamia nuts over the salad, and serve immediately.

Nutrition stats (2 cups): 218 calories, 7 g protein, 21 g carbohydrates, 13 g fat (5 g saturated), 25 mg cholesterol, 3 g fiber, 636 mg sodium.

Elisabeth Hasselbeck

Quinoa Salad

This filling salad is high in manganese, which is crucial for healthy skin and bones. Quinoa and chickpeas bring a boost of iron, needed for healthy blood.

SERVES 4

I cup quinoa, rinsed under cold running water

Grated zest and juice of I lime

2 tablespoons olive oil

½ teaspoon salt

¼ teaspoon freshly ground black pepper

I 15-ounce can chickpeas, drained and well rinsed

I ripe Hass avocado, pitted, peeled, and cubed

2 oranges, peeled, seeded, and sectioned

4 scallions, thinly sliced, using both white and green parts

½ cup fresh mint leaves, chopped

1. Place the quinoa in a small saucepan and add 2 cups of water. Bring to a simmer over medium heat; then cover and reduce the heat to low. Cook for 20 to 25 minutes, or until the quinoa is tender and the seeds are translucent in the center. Drain off any remaining liquid, and set the quinoa aside.

2. Place the lime zest and juice, olive oil, salt, and black pepper in a large salad bowl. Whisk until combined. Add the chickpeas, avocado, orange segments, quinoa, scallions, and mint. Toss gently to combine, and serve immediately.

Nutrition stats (2 cups): 472 calories, 12 g protein, 71 g carbohydrates, 16 g fat (1 g saturated), 0 mg cholesterol, 13 g fiber, 655 mg sodium.

Ruby Red Salad

Fresh, antioxidant-rich pomegranate seeds sparkle in this salad like tiny rubies. Enjoy this dish as part of your "get fit" routine or serve it as a first course for a small, cozy fall dinner party.

SERVES 4

3 large beets (about ½ pound total), or 1 15-ounce can cooked beets, drained
½ pound baby arugula
1 pomegranate, seeds removed and reserved, or 1 cup fresh pomegranate seeds
1 fennel bulb, trimmed and thinly sliced
½ small red onion, thinly sliced

Dressing
3 tablespoons olive oil
2 tablespoons sherry vinegar
1 garlic clove, cut in half
1 teaspoon salt
1 teaspoon granulated sugar
½ teaspoon dried oregano
½ cup fresh basil leaves
¼ teaspoon freshly ground black pepper
¼ cup shaved Asiago or Manchego cheese

1. *If you are using fresh beets:* Peel and quarter the beets. Fill a small saucepan about three-fourths full of water, add the beets, and simmer over medium-low heat for 45 to 50 minutes, or until they are fork-tender; drain and set aside. When the beets are cool

Elisabeth Hasselbeck

enough to handle, dice them and place them in a large bowl. *If you are using canned beets*, dice them and place them in a large bowl.

2. Add the arugula, pomegranate seeds, fennel, and onion to the beets, and toss to mix.

3. Prepare the dressing: Place the olive oil, vinegar, garlic, salt, sugar, oregano, basil, and black pepper in a blender. Process until the basil is finely chopped and the mixture is a pale green. Drizzle over the arugula mixture and toss.

4. Transfer the salad to a large platter, and arrange the cheese shavings on top. Serve immediately.

Nutrition stats (2 cups): 226 calories, 5 g protein, 22 g carbohydrates, 13 g fat (3 g saturated), 7 mg cholesterol, 6 g fiber, 752 mg sodium.

Rob the Cobb Skinny Salad

"I'll have the Cobb Salad but hold the bacon, the blue cheese, and the dressing, please." Does this sound familiar? If so, then you have just robbed the Cobb of its most flavorful ingredients (and I have been right there with you many times!). In this remake, I've given the Cobb its rightly earned flavor but managed to rob it of calories and saturated fat.

SERVES 4

¼ cup honey
3 tablespoons gluten-free Dijon mustard
1 large head romaine lettuce, thinly sliced
2 cups shredded cooked chicken
8 slices gluten-free bacon, cooked and chopped
2 Hass avocados, pitted, peeled, and cubed
2 cups corn kernels, fresh or frozen (defrosted if frozen)
2 large tomatoes, diced

1. Place the honey and the mustard in a small bowl, and add 1 tablespoon of warm water. Whisk to combine, and set aside.

2. Arrange the romaine, chicken, bacon, avocados, corn, and tomatoes on a platter. Drizzle the dressing over the top, and serve immediately.

Nutrition stats (3 cups): 351 calories, 16 g protein, 43 g carbohydrates, 13 g fat (3 g saturated), 35 mg cholesterol, 6 g fiber, 688 mg sodium.

Elisabeth Hasselbeck

Mango Salad with Lemon Chicken

Chop, chill, and serve. Your guests won't stop talking about it!

SERVES 4

Chicken

4 thin-sliced chicken cutlets (about ¾ pound total)

½ cup fresh lemon juice (from about 4 small lemons)

2 tablespoons light olive oil or canola oil

½ teaspoon salt

Dressing

3 tablespoons light olive oil or canola oil

2 tablespoons regular or creamy-style honey

2 tablespoons fresh lemon juice

½ teaspoon gluten-free Madras curry powder

Salad

10 ounces mixed salad greens or mesclun mix

2 large ripe mangoes, peeled, pitted, and chopped or sliced

½ red onion, thinly sliced

1. Place the chicken cutlets in a zipper-lock bag and add the lemon juice and 1 tablespoon of the olive or canola oil. Let marinate in the refrigerator for 1 hour.

2. Remove the chicken from the marinade and dry it with a paper towel. Sprinkle the chicken with the salt.

3. Heat a large skillet over high heat, and add the remaining 1 tablespoon oil. Add the chicken and cook, turning once, until it has browned and is cooked through, 4 to 5 minutes. Transfer to a plate.

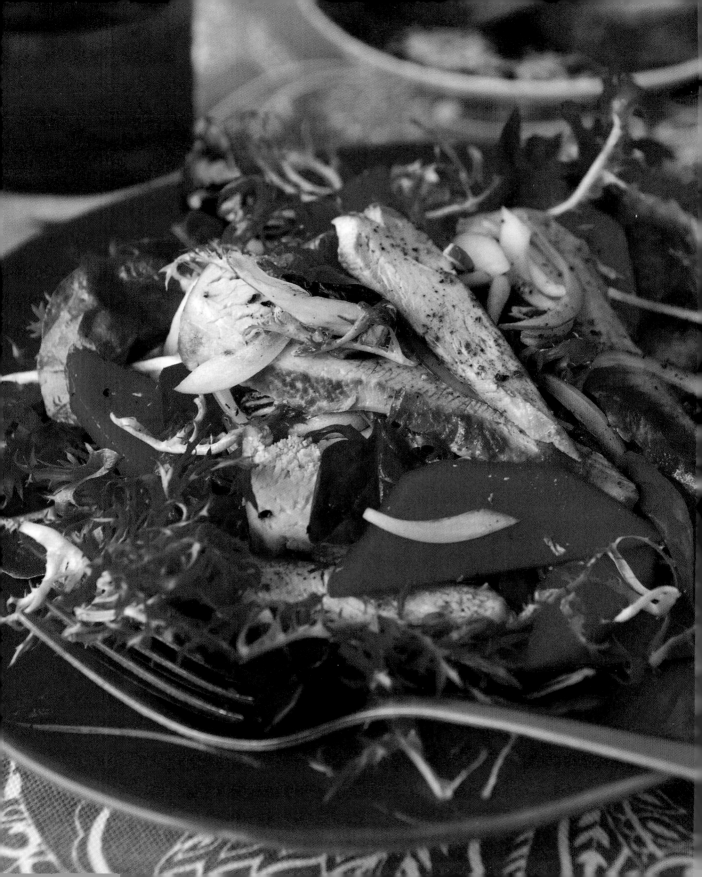

4. Make the dressing: In a small bowl, whisk the olive or canola oil, the honey, lemon juice, and curry powder together.

5. To assemble the salad, place the greens, mangoes, and onion in a large bowl or on a platter. Slice the chicken and arrange it on top of the greens. Drizzle with the dressing, and serve immediately.

Nutrition stats (3 cups): 370 calories, 20 g protein, 30 g carbohydrates, 19 g fat (2 g saturated), 7 mg cholesterol, 3 g fiber, 417 mg sodium.

{ *Acknowledgments* }

My thanks go to the incredible team at Random House and Ballantine: it has been an honor to work with you all.

To Libby McGuire, my publisher: the chance to bring *Deliciously G-Free* to the growing audience is a dream come true. Thank you for the opportunity to share what I have learned and what I love to make with my g-free community!

Marnie Cochran, a most superb editor at Ballantine, thank you for really getting this project and understanding my vision. Working alongside you has been easy and fun. Thank you for actualizing on all creative aspects . . . and for making this book as solidly informative as it is gorgeous! Your careful and keen eye has been one that I have relied upon, and I am truly grateful.

Jennifer Iserloh, you are a most gifted chef! My deep appreciation for all that you have done to work with me to create the most phenomenal g-free food I have ever made and tasted. You have taught me so much! Thank you for becoming part of our kitchen and our family. My kids loved you right from the jump; you have a most patient way with both cuisine and children. Your food is simply divine and your heart is made of gold! You are always welcome in our home, as the kitchen is a bright place when you are there.

Kelly Campbell: your artistic eye, understanding of light, and ability to capture food are astounding. Thank you for making every dish look as good as it tastes. And my sincere appreciation for catching the most precious moments of cooking with my kids. We all felt so comfortable!

Roscoe Betsil: Thank you for working as such a great team with Kelly. Everything looked divine! I so appreciate your understanding of the creative vision I had for showing off these gluten-free greats! Well done!

To my family at ABC's *The View* and *Good Morning America*—Thank you for letting me have my g-free moments. I love you all and *who knew* the *View* table would include a celiac?! Bill Geddie, many thanks for celebrating the voice of this celiac when I need to get loud about it, for the fantastic segments on awareness, and for the gluten-free cakes on my birthdays!

Barbara Walters: Thank you for all that you have done for me, in my career and in my life. There is no one better than you, and every day I learn from you. I will try to pay back my debt of gratitude with g-free chocolate bark!

Whoopi: You know I love you and so cherish our friendship. Thanks for always making sure that there is something I can eat at your home, and for making a place in your heart for me too!

Sherri: What a blessing it is to have you as my friend—you bring such light to all situations and I am thankful that we can tread through mommyland together.

Joy: I now challenge you to a lasagna contest!

To Karl Nilsson at ABC: Thank you for always looking out for me, and for all that you have done to help get the word out about my g-free-ness. You are the best of the best, and your discernment is so valued.

To all the producers, staff, and crew at *GMA* and *The View*, I love you all!

To Karen Dupiche, for the most outstanding makeup every day—but in this case, for the cover of the book. You start my days at work, and I am so happy to call you a friend. You can beat my face anytime!

To Lavette Slater, for turning the ponytail that I walk in with every day into something fantastic. Thank you!

To Caitlin May and Susan Harrington for the endless notes, schedule changes, and organizational skills without which this book would be long overdue. Thank you for energetically becoming a part of our crazy work zone, and for tackling the most ever-changing, complex calendars.

To Dr. Peter Green, MD, author of *Celiac Disease: A Hidden Epidemic*, and to Cynthia Beckman at the Celiac Disease Center in New York City: Thank you both for your pure commitment to giving celiacs their lives back. Peter, you gave me mine back for sure when I found you in NYC years ago. Thank you for your perseverance in medicine, and for your devotion to your patients. I am thankful that you are my physician, and happy to call you my friend.

To my team of agents:

To my captain and coach, Babette Perry, head of broadcasting at IMG, thank you for being with me all through the years, for walking me through career decisions, and for trusting me while at the same time nudging me to take some chances. You are a most wonderful friend and an outstanding agent. You're also an incredible mom and I will always look forward to trading family stories with you.

Andrea Barzvi, my literary agent at ICM, thank you for knowing me well, and for understanding the type of books that I love to write. Thank you for being there through it all and for endless support.

Tim Rothwell and Lisa Mitchell at IMG, two individuals who absolutely took a chance on me with my gluten-free concepts, are the best at what they do in licensing. Thank you for being by my side and for being such catalysts in the world of product, and for the fantastic commitment you have to the NoGii line.

To the NoGii team, Eric Hillman, Europa, and Shubox, my gratitude for the great job on the NoGii bars and NoGii kids' bars. The result speaks for itself, and I am proud to put out a product that I love so much. Many thanks for trusting in the g-free journey that I proposed. Ours has been a remarkable partnership.

To the entire celiac and gluten-free community: I am proud and honored to be a member. Thank you for your support, and for being the most incredible teammates in health. This book is written with you in my heart.

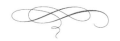

To Matthew, Sarah, Annabelle, Mallory, and Henry—thank you for making all of our visits fun and g-free!

To Don and Betsy: thank you for always having a fun selection of g-free food, for keeping a section of the grill g-free just for me, and for raising the most amazing son, my husband! I am blessed beyond mention to have you in my life.

Super Mimi, thank you for taking someone not confident with pounds of meat and making me love to prepare it now! You are beyond Super in every way. We love you so.

Grandma, Grandpa, and Mama Great: I wish you were here to taste and try, but I will think of you every time I make the feasts that you shared with us. You are always in our hearts.

Mama, how can I begin to honor you? I am forever grateful for the time that we had together as I grew up. You made me see cooking as love, not as a chore. I only wish that I had you by my side to make these g-free versions of your specialties. Each time I make meatballs, I count them just for you.

Mom, Dad, and Kenny: There are not enough words to thank you for all that you have given me. Your unconditional love and support through the years is treasured. Thank you for loving me no matter what. Thank you for carrying on the traditions of food from your families. Thank you for showing me that one can work and raise a family well. Your examples in life constantly shape and light my path. Thank you for always thinking of me, for guiding me through the most meaningful recipes in this book . . . and for ensuring that I can pass them down and continue to make great family food for Tim and the kids. I love you, always.

To Grace, Taylor, and Isaiah: I love you with my whole heart, more and more each day. Thank you for being Mommy's gluten guards. Thank you for the kindness you show one another and for all the taste-testing you did. Cooking and baking with you is my most favorite time in the kitchen. Great job! You have become the best chefs!

To my husband, Tim: My gratitude can be matched only by the love I have for you. Thank you for sitting next to me while I typed away at the text for this book and for standing up for me when I need it most. Thank you for being the most honest (thankfully, brutally honest) taste-tester I could ever ask for. This book is great for celiacs like me, but it is great for *everyone* because of you. Your insight into taste and your feedback on every dish are what made me strive to make each round better. Most important, thank you for being my best friend and my true love. With you by my side, I am strong.

{Index}

About the Author

Daytime Emmy Award winner ELISABETH HASSELBECK has been a co-host on ABC's *The View* since 2003, and in 2010 she joined ABC News and *Good Morning America* as a contributor. The author of the *New York Times* bestseller *The G-Free Diet*, she has created all-natural NoGii gluten-free protein bars for the entire family. She lives in New York City with her husband, Tim Hasselbeck, ESPN NFL analyst and former NFL quarterback, and their three children, Grace, Taylor, and Isaiah.

www.deliciouslygfree.com

About the Type

The text of this book was set in a Monotype face called Bell. The Englishman John Bell (1745–1831) was responsible for the original cutting of this design. The vocations of Bell were many—among others, bookseller, printer, publisher, type founder, and journalist. His types were considerably influenced by the delicacy and beauty of the French copper-plate engravers. Monotype Bell might also be classified as a delicate and refined rendering of Scotch Roman.